The Healing Soup Cookbook

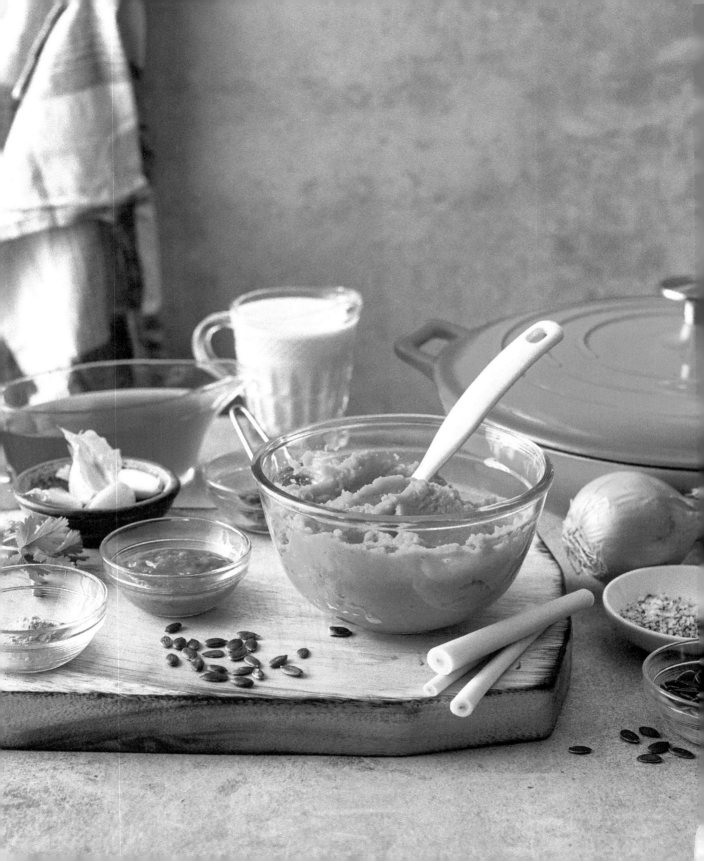

The *healing soup* Cookbook

Hearty Recipes to Boost Immunity and Restore Health

Cara Harbstreet, MS, RD, LD
and Julie Harrington, RD

Photography by Darren Muir

ROCKRIDGE
PRESS

For general information on our other products and services or to obtain technical support, please contact our Customer Care Department within the U.S. at (866) 744-2665, or outside the U.S. at (510) 253-0500.

Rockridge Press publishes its books in a variety of electronic and print formats. Some content that appears in print may not be available in electronic books, and vice versa.

Interior and Cover Designer: Antonio Valverde
Photo Art Director/Art Manager: Michael Hardgrove
Editors: Salwa Jabado and Daniel Grogan
Production Editor: Ashley Polikoff
Photography ©2019 Darren Muir. Food styling by Yolanda Muir.
Author photos courtesy of ©Cara Harbstreet: Meredith Graves Photography, ©Julie Harrington: Jessica Schaub.

ISBN: Print 978-1-64152-690-6 | eBook 978-1-64152-691-3

*Dedicated to anyone seeking
comfort and nourishment who is
willing to step into the kitchen
to create something delicious.*
Enjoy your culinary adventure!

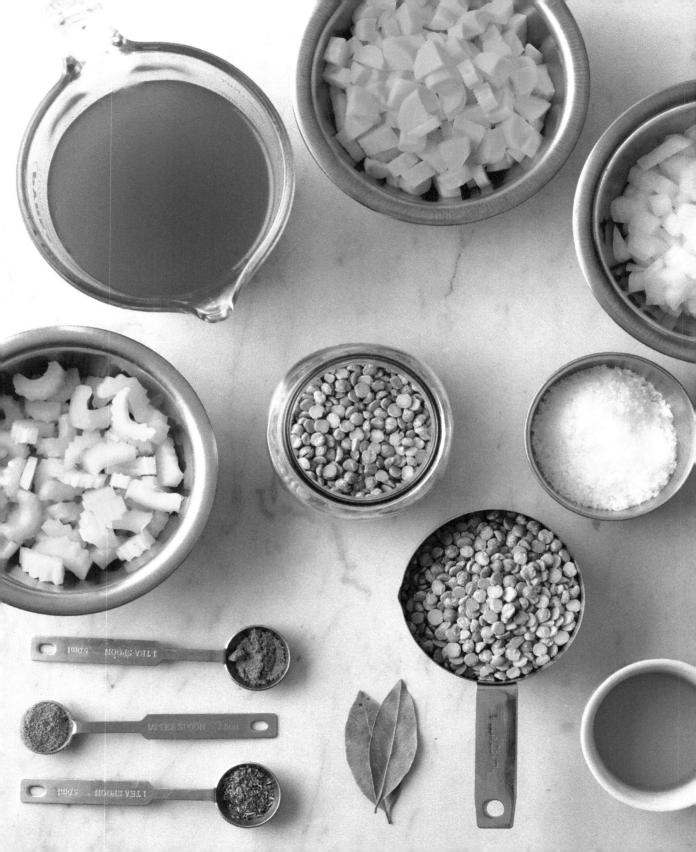

CONTENTS

4: Vegetable Soups

5: Grain and Bean Soups

6: Fish and Shellfish Soups

7: *Poultry Soups*

8: *Meaty Soups and Stews*

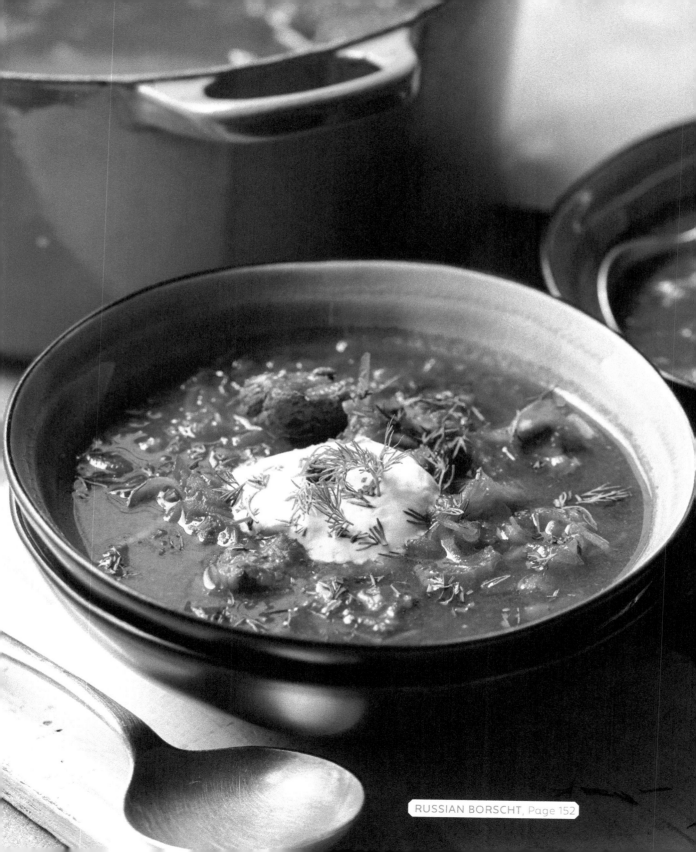

RUSSIAN BORSCHT, Page 152

INTRODUCTION

C LOSE YOUR EYES AND IMAGINE A STEAMING BOWL OF DELICIOUS SOUP. Where are you? Who are you with? How are you feeling? What do you notice about the aromas, textures, and flavors of the meal? We all probably have comforting memories that involve soups or stews, but have you ever paused to consider the power they have to heal both body and mind?

The healing power of soups and stews isn't new. In fact, cultures worldwide have embraced simple, nourishing one-pot meals for centuries. In nearly every cuisine you'll find at least a few versions of a soup that offer beneficial properties, such as Italian minestrone, Vietnamese pho, classic French onion soup, and chicken noodle soup. Some are bold and flavorful. Others are calming and mild. And though the flavors may differ across cultures, there are many common elements: Vegetables, fresh or dried herbs and spices, and savory broths and stocks create the foundation of soup that's good for the body and soul.

We created these satisfying soups so each recipe contains a balance of carbohydrates, protein, and fat from a variety of sources like vegetables, whole grains, legumes, and both plant and lean-animal proteins. Consuming a diet rich in these nutritious foods can improve energy levels, regularity, and digestion, and support a healthy immune system. You'll discover familiar favorites in this cookbook, along with new recipes that further enhance the potential for these soups and stews to replenish your body.

As dietitians who avoid strict, restrictive rules for dieting, we encourage mindful and intuitive eating because food is more than just fuel or nutrition. These soups are an opportunity to connect with family, friends, and cherished memories. We wanted to capture the soothing, satisfying feeling of being cared for with these recipes, whether you're cooking to nourish yourself or showing love for someone else when you make them.

In addition to the important emotional connection to soups and stews, we also wanted to highlight the nourishing properties of our favorite ingredients. In this modern age of hectic schedules and fewer chances to rest and recharge, it can be difficult to fight chronic, low-grade inflammation. Try as we might, it just isn't realistic to think we would never experience stress or inflammatory conditions. Our lifestyle and behaviors—including how we eat, move, and sleep; our relationships; our environment; and how much alcohol we consume—all play a role in our overall health and well-being. But you don't have to break the bank with fancy, hard to find products to take better care of yourself and your family. Simply adding more nourishing foods to your eating can offer many benefits. We've included flavorful, familiar, and affordable ingredients in these wholesome soups and stews so that they can become staples in your home cooking routine.

As two food-loving dietitians, we are grateful for this opportunity to share the warmth and love we feel in our kitchens and help you invite that same sense of healing and connection into yours. Enjoy!

Cara & Julie

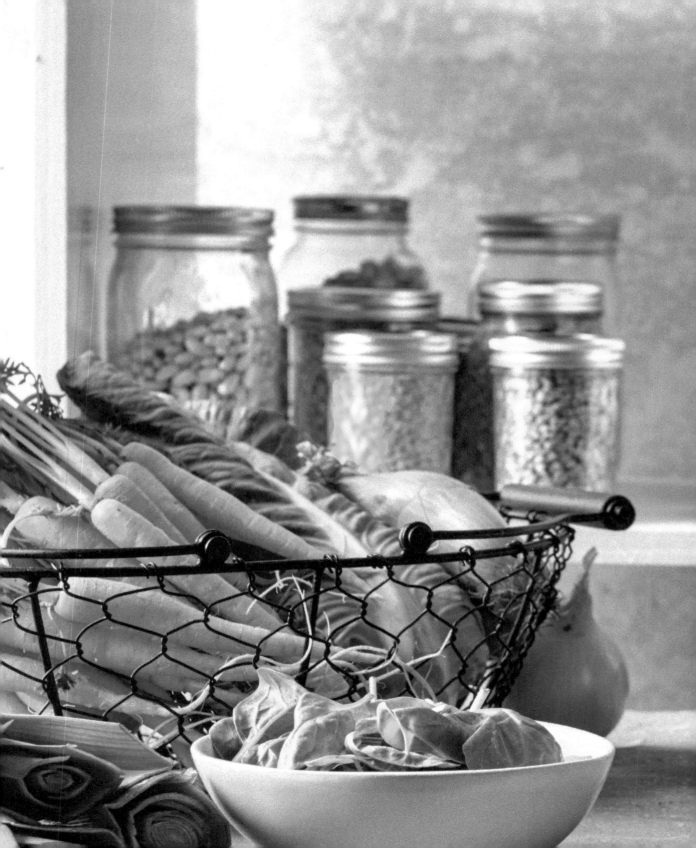

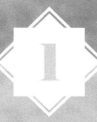

Hearty and Healthy Soups

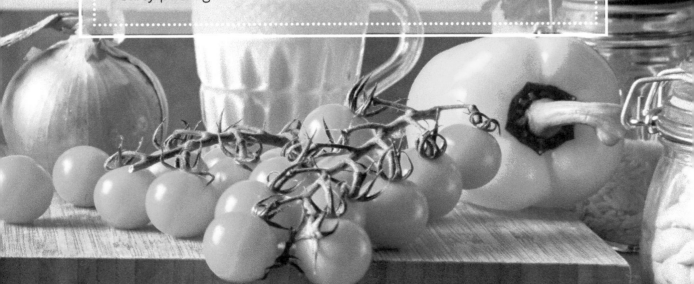

Soup is the ultimate comfort food. Whether your favorite is matzo ball, clam chowder, tomato, or another of the hundreds of soups out there, soups and stews reign supreme. They're staples around the globe for good reason—these one-pot meals provide essential nutrition, comfort, and wellness in one hearty package.

One-Pot Wellness

As two busy working professionals, we see the value in creating complete, balanced meals as conveniently as possible. Soup is one of the easiest and most versatile meals you can make. It only takes a single pot or dish, it can be made ahead, and you can adjust the recipes to suit your personal dietary needs. Americans struggle to meet the minimum daily recommendation of vegetables and fiber, and soups offer a delicious way to increase consumption of the nutrients necessary for good health.

Comfort

Soups and stews are the go-to dish when you feel less than your best. There's a simple psychological reason we tend to associate soups and stews with healing and comfort, and that's because they're often prepared by a loving parent, grandparent, or other caregiver. From the time we're very young, we understand the association between a lovingly served dish and a warm feeling of being cared for. This classical conditioning creates links in our minds to memories of how a dish makes us feel, an emotional connection that is difficult to break.

There's also a very simple physical reason why soups and stews tend to feel so comforting. Because of their high liquid content and palatable flavors, they're one of the few foods that might sound appetizing when you're feeling unwell. Soups and stews are also very easy to eat and digest because of the softer textures. This is soothing when you have a sore throat, upset tummy, or are feeling too tired to make much of an effort to eat.

But you don't have to be sick to thoroughly enjoy the comforting elements of soups! We crave these same things when we have been outside too long or are feeling chilled, want something easy to prepare that doesn't take a lot of time, or just desire the simplicity of a one-pot meal.

It's easy to see why we turn to soups and stews when we want to feel comforted or cared for. We hope these recipes become the ones you turn to when you want to care for yourself or others!

Healthy Ingredients

As dietitians, we've seen firsthand how nourishment can be a form of self-care. Food has the ability to provide essential nutrition, of course, but in addition to that, it can also offer a sense of satisfaction and delicious taste. The hallmark ingredients of a good soup or stew are typically rich in the nutrients necessary for good health:

- Vegetables rich in vitamins, minerals, and fiber
- Proteins for building deep flavor and supporting fullness and satisfaction
- Beans, legumes, and whole grains that add fiber

When combined with savory broths or stocks, you can easily create a complete meal that balances flavor and nutrition in a single bowl.

Inexpensive and Easy to Make

Anyone who's dined in a restaurant likely knows that browsing the soup section of a menu is usually gentler on your wallet. That's because the staple ingredients of soups and stews tend to be among the most affordable. Fresh herbs and vegetables can be purchased affordably in season, or we can use frozen or canned vegetables and dried/ground herbs and spices. Beans, legumes, and whole grains are among the least expensive items in a grocery store, even more so when purchased in bulk with less packaging. Added bonus: less waste!

Even the proteins we focused on for these recipes can be highly budget friendly. Soups and stews are where tougher cuts of meat get to shine thanks to the long, slow cooking process that gently heats tough proteins and yields a tender, flavorful bite.

We find inspiration in the words of the late Anthony Bourdain, a chef who loved to celebrate the flavor and culture of food. He said, "Good food is very often, even most often, simple food." So, let's keep it simple in the kitchen, with simple food prepared well.

Chicken Soup and Beyond

There's no getting around it: Chicken soup is the ultimate feel-good comfort soup in the United States.

While we certainly identify strongly with the real or perceived benefits of chicken soup, Americans aren't alone. Did you realize there are many other versions from around the world? Let's take a look at one of the most ubiquitous cross-cultural dishes.

Healing Soups around the World

- In South and Central America, you'll find *sopa del pollo* or *caldo de pollo*, a "chicken soup" that's open for interpretation, depending on the region and cuisine. It may feature potatoes, corn, or plantains and be seasoned with fresh herbs similar to cilantro.

- Matzo ball soup is served in nearly every delicatessen but is embraced outside of Jewish tradition. It's long been hailed as a cure-all and is easily recognized by the fluffy matzo balls (made from matzo meal and egg).

- In Jamaica and the Caribbean, no part of the chicken goes to waste in chicken foot soup. Chicken feet and necks are a good source of collagen, the same protein found in connective tissues like our skin, muscle, and bones. Although more research is needed to understand if food sources of collagen provide the same benefit as collagen in supplements, recipes with collagen-rich ingredients are common among cultures worldwide.

- *Samgyetang*, a Korean chicken soup, is spiced with ginseng and is cooked with a whole chicken. It's commonly served on hot summer nights. There is also *jjigae*, a broth-based stew that features the strong flavor of red pepper paste.

- Greek lemon chicken soup is made with a base of avgolemono (a sauce made with egg yolks and lemon) and includes egg, rice, celery, carrot, and onion.

This is just a small sampling of the various ways chicken soups show up in cuisines near and far, and you'll see how we drew inspiration from some of these classic dishes in the recipes for this book!

Inflammation Nation

Inflammation is a term commonly used in today's health media, but it's often misunderstood. There are two forms of inflammation:

1. **Acute** inflammation is a natural part of the body's healing process. This is what causes swelling, redness, or pain when you injure yourself or experience a temporary illness.

2. **Chronic** inflammation is ongoing low-grade inflammation that results from any number of factors. It's not noticeable in the same way as a swollen joint or painful injury, but it instead shows up as biomarkers in the blood or manifests as symptoms of chronic disease.

Here's another way to think of it: Acute inflammation is like a campfire. It burns hot and bright but only for a short period of time. It provides a purpose (to keep you warm) and can be essential and protective. Chronic inflammation is like the hot coals that remain after you think you've put the fire out. They smolder at a lower temperature and may not be as noticeable. This is where the risk lies, because there is potential for them to lead to much bigger and more serious issues over time if they aren't addressed.

An anti-inflammatory diet eating pattern is aimed to prevent or reduce low-grade chronic inflammation, a key risk factor in a host of health problems and several major diseases. While no individual meal or recipe has the power to reverse inflammation or heal one's body completely, soups and stews can provide powerful nutrition in an enjoyable way.

Common Causes of Inflammation

Inflammation is an immune response to injury or infection, and because the immune system is complex, inflammation can be triggered by our environment, genetics, or lifestyle.

We are exposed to many things in our daily life that may contribute to chronic inflammation. Factors like environmental stressors, pathogens

CULTURED AND FERMENTED FOODS

Cultured and fermented foods are easier to find than ever before, thanks to a surge in popularity. And for good reason! They may help strengthen your gut microbiome; these microorganisms are important for healthy digestion and may boost your immunity.

They can add depth of flavor to any dish, including soups and stews. The key to incorporating fermented foods such as kimchi, sauerkraut, or miso into your recipes is to allow your dish to cool to a warm, but not steaming hot, temperature. This ensures the enzymes and beneficial bacteria (probiotics) are not damaged.

or viruses, illness, stress, and trauma are part of life, whether we like it or not. They can't be avoided completely, but overly hectic lifestyles make it more challenging to combat inflammation. Lack of sleep or inconsistent self-care practices can increase stress and anxiety, and things like overexercising or underfueling your body can place it in a high-stress, inflammatory state. There's no need to feel badly about not being able to prioritize taking care of yourself all of the time, but long hours at work, minimal rest, or simply pushing your body too hard can compound the impact of stress.

It's important to point out that although our genetics may determine our predisposition for certain diseases, our lifestyle choices have the power to influence and reduce this risk, at least to some degree. When we look at healthy populations around the world, we see some commonalities among them. Things like eating a nourishing diet, engaging in enjoyable forms of movement, cultivating meaningful relationships, staying socially connected, and minimizing stress are all things that can bolster health across the lifespan. These behaviors are not unique to a diet intended to be anti-inflammatory in nature but can coexist alongside incorporating more anti-inflammatory foods.

In addition, we are learning that the gut is a critical player in immunity and total body health because many cells in the gut lining perform important functions for keeping us healthy. When the gut is functioning optimally, it may help mitigate inflammation.

Common Inflammatory Diseases

Inflammatory diseases vary in symptoms and severity, but here are some of the most common inflammatory conditions:

+ Asthma

+ Rheumatoid arthritis

+ Ulcerative colitis or Crohn's disease

+ Cardiovascular disease

+ Autoimmune conditions

+ Allergies

In addition to those listed above, chronic inflammation plays a role in other diseases such as type 2 diabetes, certain types of cancers, and other chronic or lifestyle diseases. However, it should be noted that inflammation is not something we can avoid altogether; it's a natural physiological process and our risk for many of these diseases increases with age. More research needs to be done to fully understand the complicated role that inflammation plays, but in the meantime, focusing on a diet that provides essential nutrients from a variety of foods can support health as you grow older.

How Soup Can Help

Wholesome, nutritious food is essential to good health and what we eat can play a role in minimizing inflammation and supporting anti-inflammatory pathways in the body. Soup is an enjoyable way to increase our intake of essential nutrients. We'll take a closer look at specific soup ingredients later in the chapter, but here are key elements of an anti-inflammatory diet.

OMEGA-3 FATTY ACIDS: There are two forms of this essential fatty acid found in foods such as fish and seafood, nuts and seeds, avocados, and oils. Other foods contain smaller amounts, but these fats work to slow inflammatory pathways and combat inflammation in the body.

POLYPHENOLS AND ANTIOXIDANTS: This broad category of compounds does not contribute calories to our diets, but it does provide other essential things for our bodies. Polyphenols (also sometimes called phytochemicals or polyphenolic compounds) are abundant in plant foods. There are over 8,000 identified polyphenols that can be a source of dietary antioxidants. Antioxidants help combat damage from free radicals (which can contribute to overall inflammation) and support overall health.

FIBER: Most Americans aren't consuming enough fiber. Ingredients in soups and stews, namely vegetables, can contribute both soluble and insoluble fiber to our diets, supporting better gut health along with keeping us feeling full. The microbiome plays an important role in immunity and overall health, and adding more fiber to your diet can help.

Building Soup

You may have been in a rush to put dinner on the table and attempted the "toss in anything about to spoil and hope for the best" approach to cooking soups and stews. And in a pinch, that can work, but there are ways to be more strategic about building delicious flavor for a better eating experience.

BASE: The base is the foundation of a soup, made up of a flavorful stock or broth. The recipes we feature in chapter 2 will provide the essence of your recipe and pull from various cuisines, from classic French cooking to Asian-inspired flavors to trendy bone broth.

AROMATICS: Aromatics is just a fancy term for bold and fragrant vegetables. The most common aromatics are mirepoix, a French term for the classic combination of onions, carrots, celery, and sometimes leeks. Most often garlic is added to the classic mirepoix. Or the Cajun "holy trinity" consists of red bell pepper, onions, and celery. Aromatics are essentials to begin the process of building the flavors of a soup.

VEGETABLES: Nearly any vegetable can be turned into a tasty, healthy soup, but knowing the properties of each vegetable is key—like understanding its taste profile, cook time, and what it will pair well with. For example, chopped butternut squash needs to be added to a soup earlier in the cooking process than kale because they have different cook times, and vegetables like onions will have an enhanced flavor if allowed to caramelize.

BROTHS: TO MAKE OR TO BUY

There's nothing wrong with choosing to purchase a premade stock or broth at the grocery store, but some people prefer to make their own at home. Both will serve the same purpose of giving you a flavorful liquid from which to build the rest of your recipe. If you're on the fence, remember a few key things:

COST: It may be less expensive to use the recipes in chapter 2 to create batches of broths and stocks at home. Going this route can also help you use up scraps from your kitchen, stretching your grocery budget further and reducing food waste. If purchasing from the grocery store, expect to pay a little bit more per serving compared to homemade.

CONVENIENCE: It can be a gratifying experience to prepare a stock or broth from scratch. However, if you're short on time, you may find it easier to purchase instead.

FLAVOR: Our perception of flavor is unique to each of us, and you won't know your true taste preferences until you experiment. There is a wide variety of stocks and broths on the market today, including bone broths and those with unique seasonings or flavor profiles. Another thing to be aware of is the varying sodium levels. There can be a drastic difference between store-bought and homemade, but salt alone doesn't build deep flavor. If you're unsure whether your palate can discern a difference, try preparing the same recipe on different nights with each version. Taste-testing like this can help you learn what to rely on for future recipes.

NUTRITIONAL VALUE: Aside from differences in sodium content, it can be challenging to identify a significant difference between the nutritional value of a store-bought broth or stock compared to homemade. However, if you have known food allergies or sensitivities, you may prefer to prepare your own versions to avoid ingredients that may trigger GI symptoms.

PROTEINS (OPTIONAL): No matter your preference for plant- or animal-based proteins, there are myriad options. Depending on the cooking method, you can add proteins early in the cooking process (for example, when using a tougher cut of meat or relying on dry beans or legumes for plant-based protein) or late in the game (like with thawed, pre-cooked shrimp or seafood with a delicate texture). Most proteins hold up well when immersed in the liquid of a soup or stew, but be mindful of food safety, regardless of where you choose to source your protein.

TOPPERS: This can be the most fun part of serving soups and stews! Get creative and adventurous with your bowl toppers and experiment with flavors and textures. A common strategy is to finish with fresh herbs. Don't add fresh herbs too early on during the cooking process, as their delicate aromas will cook away. Other options include crispy chickpeas, nuts or seeds, ground spices or other seasonings, and shredded cheese or sour cream for a creamier texture.

Soup Lover's Pantry

Stocking your pantry to prepare delicious home-cooked soups doesn't need to be a major process. In fact, you likely already have many of the basic ingredients in your kitchen right now. We wrote these recipes with flexibility in mind. They are meant to be adjusted according to your taste preferences, availability of ingredients, and budget. We suggest browsing through the recipes first to see what looks interesting, then taking stock of your pantry, fridge, and freezer before shopping. This strategy can help you avoid duplicate purchases and reduce food waste.

Nourishing Basics

These ingredients make up the bulk of a soup or stew. They contribute the basic flavors and textures, as well as basic nutrition from carbohydrates, fats, and proteins.

ONIONS: Onions are readily available year-round and make an affordable, convenient option for adding flavor and bulk to soups and stews. They can also be purchased frozen or prechopped if you're not inclined to tackle that task yourself!

CARROTS: Carrots are another essential basic. They add a subtle sweetness and pop of color, and they can be cooked to varying textures to enhance the overall recipe.

CELERY: When combined with onions and carrots, celery becomes the third key ingredient for a classic mirepoix. This aromatic combination, originating in French cooking and cuisine, serves as a flavor base for soups, stews, sauces, and more.

BROTH: Whether a thin soup or a thick, hearty stew, cooking with a broth or stock adds more flavor to your recipe than simply using water for the liquid component. Make your own (see chapter 2) or purchase a flavorful broth (see page 9 for tips).

BEANS: Canned beans are another affordable, easy-to-find ingredient that requires little to no prep. If cooking from dried, be aware you'll need to account for additional prep time for soaking and cooking.

POTATOES: Potatoes are another inexpensive, versatile base ingredient for many soups. Potatoes of all varieties, including white, baby/new, purple, red, yellow, and sweet potatoes, contribute energizing carbohydrates, vitamins, minerals, and fiber.

HERBS AND SPICES: These build upon the base of flavor created with other ingredients and your stock or broth. Some of our favorites include garlic, ginger, cumin, paprika, parsley, rosemary, oregano, and chives. You can add them toward the beginning or the end of cooking depending on whether you use fresh or dried. Create the flavor profile you like best!

Healing Flavor Enhancers

To build upon nourishing basics, you can add additional ingredients to enhance flavor and further support health.

GARLIC: Sulfuric compounds in garlic are associated with anti-inflammatory properties. Thankfully its flavor pairs well with many ingredients so there is ample opportunity to include it in recipes.

TURMERIC WITH BLACK PEPPER: There is a great deal of research investigating the role of turmeric for health, especially the curcumin

A NOTE ABOUT NIGHTSHADES

Arthritis and joint pain are two of the most common examples of inflammation in the body. Anyone who has experienced this firsthand knows it can range from discomfort that is slightly annoying to debilitating pain. And despite one's best efforts to treat or manage symptoms, relief is sometimes difficult to find. Many people turn their focus to their diet in an effort to identify potential triggers among the foods they eat.

One food group in particular that has received criticism as a contributor to inflammation is nightshade vegetables. Botanically speaking, nightshades are members of the Solanaceae family. The name derives from solanine, an alkaloid compound that serves to protect the plant. The most common nightshade vegetables are tomatoes, bell peppers, potatoes, okra, and eggplants, but there are over 2,000 species within this botanical family. Spices such as paprika and cayenne pepper are also included because they are sourced from peppers.

While some people are sensitive to solanine and may notice their symptoms are exacerbated when they consume nightshade vegetables, there are no scientific studies suggesting that nightshades promote inflammation. Not everyone with arthritis experiences worsened symptoms, so there is no reason to avoid them if you have not noticed symptoms as a result of eating them. Solanine is more highly concentrated in the leaves and stems of plants rather than the edible parts that we usually consume. Not only that, but these nightshade vegetables provide important nutrients and polyphenols that may actually help combat inflammation. That's why we have included them in so many of the recipes in this cookbook.

The bottom line: It is safe to enjoy nightshade vegetables!

compound. Absorption is enhanced significantly when consumed with black pepper (due to the pepperin compound), so remember to pair the two together for optimal absorption.

GINGER: Ginger is commonly used in cultures worldwide for treating gastrointestinal ailments, nausea, joint pain, and more. In addition to soups and stews, you may find it in certain beverages or baked items.

CINNAMON: While commonly thought of as a sweet flavor pairing, cinnamon can add depth and richness to savory dishes as well. You'll find cinnamon in spice blends or Indian or Thai curry, but you can openly experiment with adding small amounts to enhance flavor in any type of dish. Cinnamon is being researched as an anti-inflammatory tool that could potentially aide in blood sugar management.

OLIVE OIL: Olive oil is a rich source of anti-inflammatory omega-3 fatty acids. It generally has a mild flavor, so it's ideal for sautéing or roasting ingredients that end up in your soup or stew.

NUTS: Another source of omega-3 fatty acids and fiber, nuts can add an appetizing texture to soups and stews. Look for them in some of our recipes for blended soups (among others) to make the smooth texture more filling.

LEAFY GREENS: While fresh leafy greens may only be available seasonally, frozen options are available year-round. They can be seamlessly and easily incorporated into soups and stews to enhance both flavor and nutrition. Kale and spinach are two that work particularly well in these recipes, but watercress or chard could be interesting substitutions.

Kitchen Tools and Equipment

The recipes that follow in the next chapters are simple to make, but as with any cooking, the right tools for the job will make these so much easier to prepare.

Must-Have

STOCKPOT: Stockpots are typically larger than a regular large pot. The tall sides prevent too much liquid from evaporating during long cooking times. Their size also allows you to prepare larger batches of your recipe if you wish, leaving you with extra portions to enjoy as leftovers or to freeze for later. For the recipes in this book, an eight- to twelve-quart stockpot will do the trick.

LONG-HANDLED WOODEN SPOON: Make sure the wooden spoon can reach the bottom of your pot. A wooden spoon stays cool and can easily scrape any bits stuck on the bottom of the pot.

LADLE: Transfer soup to a bowl or storage container with a deep, round-bottom ladle. Opt for stainless steel if you can, as heat-safe plastic ladles have potential BPA concerns, and might melt if the stovetop gets too hot.

CUTTING BOARDS AND KNIFE SET: These tools go hand in hand and are truly essential because you'll find yourself reaching for them for nearly every recipe in this cookbook! If possible, stock up on more than one cutting board if you cook with raw proteins; this will limit cross-contamination. And as for knives, no need to invest in an entire block's worth; a sharpened chef's knife and paring knife will cover all your basic needs.

IMMERSION BLENDER: This tool helps you blend directly in the pot, which is far less messy than transferring batches of hot soup into a blender to purée. Plus, most immersion blenders' blades are now easily removed and dishwasher safe for easy cleanup. They are also more affordable when compared to high-speed blenders.

SOUP SKIMMER: This handheld circular strainer is great for removing unwanted froth or bits that float to the surface. You can also use it when preparing stocks or broths as needed, keeping your fingers safely away from extra-hot liquids.

Nice to Have

DUTCH OVEN: These heavy, thick-walled pots are the cast iron skillets of soup making. They come preseasoned so you don't need to worry about that step, but they allow you to brown proteins or caramelize onions in the same pot as your finished dish and build even more flavor into your recipe.

HIGH-SPEED BLENDER: Although these kitchen appliances are a bit of an investment, they are the gold standard for creating ultra-creamy and smooth soups. You'll see a few recipes that call for this tool, but if you don't have one, just use your standard blender or an immersion blender (just be aware the texture may be slightly different).

ELECTRIC PRESSURE COOKER OR SLOW COOKER: You may have noticed the electric pressure cooker craze and wondered if you should snag one of your own. It can be a convenient time-saver, but the recipes written for this cookbook can be prepared on the stovetop. Slow cookers are another useful appliance, so look for our tips in the instructions that let you know if the directions are different for this cooking method.

GLASS STORAGE CONTAINERS: When it comes to leftovers, having enough storage containers with matching lids is half the battle! We prefer the glass versions because they won't warp if you're in a rush and need to transfer hot soup into them. They also tend to have locking lids so there's less of a chance of spilling if they get knocked over. Consider investing in a set with multiple sizes so you have a variety of storage options.

Storage Tools and Tips

We are big fans of leftovers! Soups are simple to reheat on the stovetop or in the microwave, and, when stored properly, they retain both their nutritive quality and flavor. Make big batches of soup on the weekend to save valuable time and energy on busy days. Storage may seem like a no-brainer, but to avoid bacterial growth or contamination, here are a few things to keep in mind.

COOLING DOWN: Stir soup to release the heat. The FDA recommends a two-stage cooling process. Cool food from 140°F to 70°F within two hours, then to below 41°F in an additional four hours. You may also expedite the process by transferring soups and stews out of the large pot it was cooked in. This not only helps dissipate heat, but also speeds the cooling process when soup is transferred to shallow dishes that can then be cooled in an ice bath.

REFRIGERATION: Placing hot leftovers in the refrigerator can impair its cooling ability. Try to allow foods to cool adequately (up to two hours) before placing in your fridge and be sure to avoid packing or stacking your storage containers too tightly. When there is room for air to circulate above, below, and around storage containers, soup leftovers will chill to a safe temperature more quickly and easily and pose less of a threat for food safety issues. Soup can be stored in the refrigerator for three to four days.

CONTAINERS: A freezer-safe plastic or silicone bag can help you save space in your freezer. To pour soup in a bag, place the bag in a bowl and cuff the bag over the edges. Ladle cooled soup into each bag, let out excess air, and seal. Lay bags flat in a single layer in the freezer. When completely frozen, stack them.

GLASS JARS: Ensure soup is cooled properly before storing in glass jars to chill or freeze. Leave two inches on the top of the jar before securing the lid. Soup will expand as it freezes, which can result in the jar cracking or shattering during the freezing process if you do not leave enough head space at the top of the jar. Utilize glass mason jars or reuse glass pasta sauce jars (just be sure to clean them thoroughly first).

LABELS AND USE-BY DATES: Leftovers can start to look very similar once they're sealed and packed away in the fridge or freezer. Avoid confusion by creating an organized system of labeling. Name your recipe, then include both the date it was prepared and the date it should be used by. Properly stored in the freezer, soup will maintain best quality for about four to six months. Periodically go through and remove items past their "use-by" date to keep your freezer organized. Use the "first in, first out" method and make an effort to use the oldest items first (reducing food waste by ensuring things get consumed before their "use-by" date passes).

WHEN TO SKIP THE FREEZER

Freezer-friendly options may be lifesavers for hectic weeks where cooking from scratch isn't an option. But some soups are better suited for this strategy than others. There is a high likelihood that the texture of ingredients in your soups and stews will expand and change when thawing and reheating, so be aware of these ingredients that tend to perform poorly in the freezer:

LEAFY GREENS: Although they are wilted/cooked for inclusion in soup, leafy greens historically do not fare well with wide temperature fluctuations. You may notice them disintegrating when thawing and reheating, and while you won't necessarily lose out on nutrition, the texture and appearance of your recipe may suffer.

RICE-BASED SOUPS: Soups that feature rice are not ideal for freezing. Because of the high starch content, the rice tends to absorb excess liquid and could potentially disintegrate when thawing and reheating. A better strategy? Try freezing just the soup portion then serving with freshly cooked rice when you're ready to enjoy it.

TOFU: When it comes to proteins, most will fare well in the freezer and face few issues when thawing and reheating. However, because of the soft, delicate texture of tofu, you may find that it doesn't stand up quite as well.

We've highlighted several freezer-friendly soups and stews. Be on the lookout for the label indicating recipes that are great to stock your freezer.

Thawing and Reheating Soup

Food safety doesn't end with cooling food, it also matters for thawing and reheating. We recommend thawing frozen soups in the refrigerator overnight (the same can be done with premade broths or stocks before you begin cooking). Once the consistency is mostly liquefied again, you can reheat in a saucepan over medium-low heat, stirring occasionally.

Soup can be reheated in the microwave as well. Start by heating in 20- to 30-second increments, then pause to stir the contents. This helps you avoid "hot spots" of overheated soup and ensures an even temperature.

Don't be fearful of losing nutrients when using a microwave; despite a persistent myth that microwaved food is "less healthy," the reality is that all reheating methods have the potential to deactivate enzymes in food or alter nutrients. Heat is one of the primary elements that will denature proteins, but water content and length of cooking are also factors. Ironically, soups and stews by nature have a combination of high water content (moist cooking methods), long cooking times, and high temperatures. The bottom line: They still offer a healthy way to eat and microwaved food is safe to consume.

About the Recipes

And now for the fun part! As we start to explore the different categories of soups and stews, we'll start with the basics of broths and stocks from scratch in chapter 2. From there, we'll explore some traditional favorites before moving into other chapters based on their main ingredients—vegetables, grains and beans, fish and shellfish, poultry, and meat. Look for the recipe labels that indicate the types of recipes you're particularly interested in. You will find labels for:

- ◆ Gluten-Free
- ◆ Dairy-Free
- ◆ Vegetarian or Vegan
- ◆ Quick Prep
- ◆ Fast (start to finish in 30 minutes or less)
- ◆ Freezer Friendly

Each chapter will list recipes in order from puréed or blended soups to those that are heartier and more filling. All of our recipes were designed with health, nutrition, and flavor in mind. Compared to other versions of these soups, the vegetable content is higher, and we are mindful of the amount of sodium, added sugar, and saturated fat. We've also included helpful tips for ingredient swaps, flavor boosters, time-saving tricks, and other suggestions that make the cooking process more enjoyable.

You will also find per serving nutritional analysis to identify the soups that fit with your dietary needs. Please note that while nutrition information is calculated to be as accurate as possible based on the recipes as they are written, homemade stocks and broths can vary in their nutrition content, so we omitted the analysis for most of the base recipes in chapter 2.

Are you ready to get started? Let's head to the kitchen!

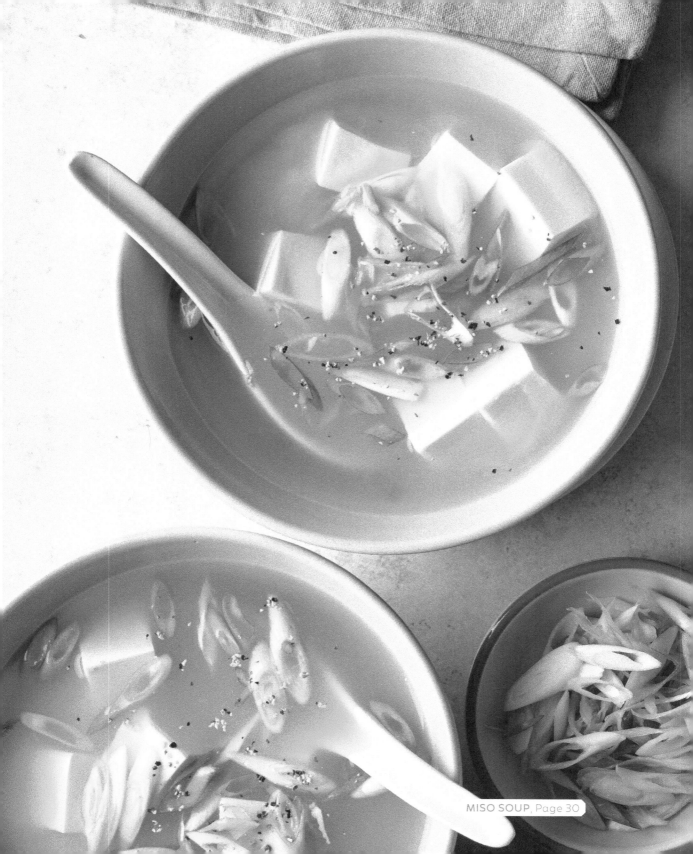

MISO SOUP, Page 30

2

Stocks and Broths

The foundation of any great soup or stew is a flavorful broth or stock. Often the terms stock and broth are used interchangeably, but there are three important differences: ingredients, cook time, and seasoning. Stock is made by simmering a combination of bones, mirepoix (carrots, celery, and onion), and aromatics in water for two to six hours. Gelatin from the bones is an essential part of stock that is created when the connective tissue in meat breaks down, giving stock its body; the gelatin is what causes stock to gel when chilled. Broth is typically made by simmering meat, mirepoix, and aromatics for a shorter amount of time, typically between one and two hours. It is also often more heavily seasoned than stock. Bone broth is a hybrid of broth and stock. It is cooked for a long period of time, and the goal is not only to extract the gelatin from the bones (like in a stock) but also to release the nutritious compounds and minerals (namely collagen, but also glucosamine, amino acids, electrolytes, calcium, and more). In this chapter, you'll find nine recipes for everything from mushroom broth to classic chicken stock. Keep these handy as they are the base of all the soups and stews in this book.

Classic Vegetable Broth

SERVES 12 | PREP TIME 15 MINUTES | **COOK TIME** 1½ HOURS

Making a classic vegetable broth is incredibly simple: Chop some vegetables, cover with water, and simmer. Why bother buying it at the store? Use this broth as the base for other soup recipes or to add flavor to other dishes. The real benefit of this recipe is the gut-healing properties of onions, leeks, and garlic. Onions and garlic are particularly rich in soluble fibers called fructans, which support a healthy microbiome.

FREEZER FRIENDLY,
GLUTEN-FREE, VEGAN,
DAIRY-FREE

1 tablespoon olive oil

2 large onions, chopped
    into 1-inch pieces

4 large carrots, peeled and
    chopped into 1-inch pieces

4 celery stalks, chopped
    into 1-inch pieces

1 leek, quartered
    and chopped

6 garlic cloves, halved

2 thyme sprigs

2 bay leaves

2 teaspoons whole
    black peppercorns

4 quarts water

Salt

1. In a large stockpot, heat the olive oil over medium-high heat. Add the onions, carrots, celery, and leek. Sauté until the onions become translucent and the vegetables are tender, 5 to 7 minutes.

2. Add the garlic, thyme, bay leaves, and black peppercorns.

3. Add the water to submerge the vegetables in the pot. (Use more, as needed.) Bring to a boil; reduce the heat and simmer until the broth is reduced by half, 1 to 1½ hours.

4. Remove the broth from the heat and let cool slightly. Strain the broth through a fine-mesh strainer into a large bowl; discard the solids.

5. Season with salt to taste.

Storage tip: Refrigerate in an airtight container for up to 1 week. Freeze for up to 3 months.

Substitution tip: You can use leftover vegetable pieces to create this broth instead of whole vegetables. When you cook, save your vegetable scraps (onion peels and ends, carrot peels, celery ends, etc.) and store in a zip-top bag in the freezer until you are ready to make the broth.

Flavor boost: Try other vegetables and herbs (such as fennel, mushrooms, rosemary, or parsley) to enhance the flavor.

Immune-Boosting Vegetable Broth

SERVES 12 | **PREP TIME** 15 MINUTES | **COOK TIME** 1 HOUR 40 MINUTES

This soothing vegan broth is enhanced with flavorful anti-inflammatory and healing herbs and spices. Turmeric's active compound, curcumin, has been extensively studied for its disease-fighting potential and health benefits. Ginger contains phenolic compounds called gingerols that exhibit many health benefits. It is anti-inflammatory, antioxidant, antimicrobial, and antiemetic (meaning it can reduce nausea), and it promotes good digestion.

FREEZER FRIENDLY,
GLUTEN-FREE, VEGAN,
DAIRY-FREE

1 tablespoon olive oil

1 large onion, chopped
   into 1-inch pieces

2 large carrots, peeled and
   chopped into 1-inch pieces

2 parsnips, peeled and
   chopped into 1-inch pieces

3 celery stalks, chopped

½ green cabbage
   head, chopped

6 garlic cloves, halved

1 parsley bunch

1 (3-inch) piece fresh ginger,
   peeled and chopped

1 tablespoon ground
   turmeric

1 teaspoon whole black
   peppercorns

4 quarts water

Salt

1. In a large stockpot, heat the olive oil over medium-high heat. Add the onions, carrots, parsnips, celery, and cabbage. Sauté until the onions become translucent and the vegetables are tender, 5 to 7 minutes.

2. Add the garlic, parsley, ginger, turmeric, and black peppercorns.

3. Add the water to submerge the vegetables in the pot. (Use more, as needed.) Bring to a boil; reduce the heat and simmer until broth is reduced by half, 1 to 1½ hours.

4. Remove the broth from the heat and let cool slightly. Strain broth through a fine-mesh strainer into a large bowl; discard the solids.

5. Season with salt to taste.

Ingredient tip: Skip the vegetable peeler when peeling ginger. Use a stainless-steel spoon and scrape off the skin with ease.

Substitution tip: Replace fresh ginger with ½ tablespoon ground ginger, if that is what you have on hand. Ginger has been known to reduce nausea or upset stomach.

Chicken Broth

SERVES 12 | PREP TIME 10 MINUTES | **COOK TIME** 2 HOURS

This delicious broth is made with anti-inflammatory vegetables, herbs, spices, and chicken. It can be enjoyed as is or used as a foundation for other soup recipes. Chicken broth contains magnesium, known as the relaxation mineral. Getting magnesium through food helps your body absorb more of it, promoting a better night's sleep.

FREEZER FRIENDLY,
GLUTEN-FREE,
DAIRY-FREE,QUICKPREP

1 (4-pound) whole chicken,
  giblets removed

2 large onions, quartered

3 carrots, peeled and cut
  into 2-inch pieces

3 celery stalks, cut into
  2-inch pieces

1 leek, halved and chopped
  into 2-inch pieces

10 garlic cloves, halved

2 bay leaves

2 or 3 thyme sprigs

1 parsley bunch

½ tablespoon whole
  black peppercorns

16 cups water

Salt

1. In a large stockpot, combine the chicken, onions, carrots, celery, leek, garlic, bay leaves, thyme, parsley, and black peppercorns. Add the water, fully submerging the ingredients. Use more if necessary.

2. Bring to a boil, then reduce to a gentle simmer. Cook for about 1 hour, until the chicken is cooked through (to 165°F). During the cooking process, skim any fat or foam that rises to the surface.

3. Remove the chicken from the broth and continue to simmer the broth with the vegetables for an additional 1 hour, again skimming any fat or foam that rises to the surface.

4. Let the chicken slightly cool and remove the meat from the bones. Reserve the chicken meat for another use.

5. Remove the pot from the heat and let cool slightly. Strain the broth through a fine-mesh strainer and discard the solids.

6. Season with salt to taste.

Substitution tip: Don't have a whole chicken? Use a combination of chicken parts: breasts, thighs, wings, and drumsticks.

Flavor boost: For different flavor variations, add other vegetables into the broth base, like parsnips, turnips, etc.

Chicken Stock

SERVES 12 | PREP TIME 10 MINUTES | **COOK TIME** 4 HOURS

Similar to a chicken broth, chicken stock just uses the bones of the chicken and simmers for a longer period of time to create a richer flavor. Because of the naturally occurring collagen and gelatin in chicken stock, eating or drinking it regularly can relieve joint pain that comes from getting older.

FREEZER FRIENDLY,
GLUTEN-FREE,
QUICK PREP

Bones from 4-pound
   chicken, including neck
   and back bones

2 large onions, quartered

3 carrots, peeled and cut
   into 2-inch pieces

3 celery stalks, cut into
   2-inch pieces

1 leek, halved and chopped
   into 2-inch pieces

10 garlic cloves, halved

2 bay leaves

2 or 3 thyme sprigs

1 parsley bunch

½ tablespoon whole
   black peppercorns

16 cups water

Salt

Black pepper

1. In a large stockpot, combine the chicken bones, onions, carrots, celery, leek, garlic, bay leaves, thyme, parsley, and black peppercorns. Add the water, fully submerging the ingredients. Use more if necessary.

2. Bring to a boil, then reduce to a simmer. Simmer for 2 to 4 hours. During the cooking process, skim any fat or foam that rises to the surface. Add hot water, as needed, to keep the bones and vegetables submerged.

3. Remove the pot from the heat and let cool slightly. Strain the stock through a fine-mesh strainer and discard the solids.

4. Season with salt and pepper to taste.

Ingredient tip: Purchase a fully cooked rotisserie chicken at the grocery store. Use the chicken for other dishes and save the bones to create this stock.

Flavor boost: Use this stock to add flavor to other recipes. For example, instead of using water to cook quinoa, use chicken stock.

Beef Stock

SERVES 8 | **PREP TIME** 20 MINUTES | **COOK TIME** 4 HOURS 40 MINUTES

Roasting the bones and vegetables in the oven first gives a hearty flavor to this basic beef stock. In addition to soups, you can use this beefy broth in stews, gravies, sauces, and vegetable dishes. The minerals and amino acids in beef stock are highly bioavailable nutrients—meaning they come in an easy-to-digest form.

FREEZER FRIENDLY,
DAIRY-FREE,
GLUTEN-FREE

5 pounds beef bones and trimmings (preferably from beef shank and short ribs)

2 medium onions, quartered

3 medium carrots, peeled and cut into 2-inch pieces

3 celery stalks, cut into 2-inch pieces

2 tablespoons olive oil

Salt

Black pepper

2 tablespoons tomato paste

12 cups water, divided

2 bay leaves

1 small parsley bunch

½ teaspoon whole black peppercorns

1 thyme sprig (or ¼ teaspoon dried thyme)

1. Preheat the oven to 400°F. In a large roasting pan, combine the bones, onions, carrots, and celery. Toss with the olive oil and season with salt and pepper. Roast for 40 minutes, stirring contents halfway through the cooking time.

2. In a large stockpot, bring 2 cups of water to a simmer. Whisk in the tomato paste until fully dissolved.

3. Add the bones and roasted vegetables, scraping any bits from the pan and juices that have accumulated. Add the remaining 10 cups of water until the bones and vegetables are fully submerged.

4. Add the bay leaves, parsley, black peppercorns, and thyme.

5. Bring to a boil and then reduce to a simmer and cook for 3 to 4 hours, skimming off any foam or fat that accumulates at the top.

6. Remove the pot from the heat and let cool slightly. Strain the stock through a fine-mesh strainer and discard the solids. Season with salt to taste.

Flavor boost: The acid from the tomato paste helps break down cartilage on the beef bones and also adds color to the finished beef stock.

Bone Broth

SERVES 8 | **PREP TIME** 15 MINUTES | **COOK TIME** 9 HOURS

The longer this nourishing broth cooks, the more concentrated the flavor becomes. Known for its healing benefits, bone broth can be enjoyed as is or as the base of other soups. Bone broth is also rich in electrolytes such as sodium, potassium, and magnesium which are essential for daily function and replenishment when you are sick.

GLUTEN-FREE, FREEZER
FRIENDLY, DAIRY-FREE

4 pounds beef marrow bones

2 large carrots, peeled and
　　cut into 2-inch pieces

1 leek, cut into 2-inch pieces

1 medium onion, quartered

8 garlic cloves

3 celery stalks, cut into
　　2-inch pieces

3 bay leaves

2 tablespoons whole
　　black peppercorns

1 tablespoon apple　·
　　cider vinegar

12 cups water

Salt

1. Preheat the oven to 450°F. In a large roasting pan, place the bones, carrots, leek, onion, and garlic. Roast for 40 minutes, stirring contents halfway through the cooking time.

2. In a large stockpot, add the bones and roasted vegetables, scraping any bits from the pan and juices that have accumulated. Add the celery, bay leaves, black peppercorns, and vinegar. Add the water (more if needed) until the contents are completely submerged.

3. Cover the pot with a lid and bring to a boil. Reduce the heat to a gentle simmer and cook with the lid slightly ajar to let out some steam. Cook for at least 8 hours (or up to 24 hours), skimming off any foam or fat that may rise to the top. Do not leave the pot unattended.

4. Add more water as necessary, ensuring the bones and vegetables are fully submerged.

5. Remove the pot from the heat and let cool slightly. Discard the bones and strain the broth through a fine-mesh strainer and discard the solids.

6. Season with salt to taste.

Continued

Ingredient tip: Beef marrow bones can be found in your local grocery store or at a butcher. Glucosamine (a natural compound found in cartilage) from the marrow in the bone broth is being studied for its potential to help repair damaged joints and reduce pain and inflammation.

Ingredient tip: The acid from the apple cider vinegar helps extract the nourishing marrow from the beef bones.

Substitution tip: For chicken bone broth, use chicken bones instead of beef bones.

Mushroom Broth

SERVES 6 | PREP TIME 15 MINUTES | **COOK TIME** 1 HOUR 15 MINUTES

This deeply flavorful broth is excellent in soups, stews, and sauces or to serve in a mug for a warm and savory beverage. This plant-powered broth has nutritional benefits, helping to improve gut health and boost the immune system.

VEGAN, FREEZER
FRIENDLY, DAIRY-FREE

3 tablespoons olive oil

2 pounds cremini
  mushrooms, finely
  chopped

½ large onion, chopped

3 garlic cloves, chopped

8 cups water

¼ cup low-sodium soy sauce

½ cup dried mushrooms,
  such as porcini or shiitake

3 thyme sprigs

Salt

1. In a large pot, heat the olive oil over medium-high heat. Add the mushrooms, onion, and garlic. Cook, stirring, until the mushrooms release their liquid, 5 to 7 minutes.

2. Add the water, soy sauce, dried mushrooms, and thyme. Stir to combine and bring to a boil.

3. Reduce the heat to a simmer, cover, and let simmer for 1 hour.

4. Pour the broth through a fine-mesh strainer. Season with salt to taste.

Ingredient tip: Mushrooms are the only source of vitamin D in the produce aisle and one of the few natural food sources. Vitamin D helps build and maintain strong bones by helping the body absorb calcium.

Substitution tip: For a gluten-free version, use a gluten-free soy sauce alternative like tamari.

Miso Soup

SERVES 6 | PREP TIME 10 MINUTES | **COOK TIME** 20 MINUTES

You've likely enjoyed miso soup out at a restaurant, but it's surprisingly easy to make at home. The Japanese ingredient miso, a fermented paste traditionally made from soybeans and sea salt, simmers to create a rich, savory broth.

FAST, GLUTEN-FREE,
QUICK PREP, VEGAN,
DAIRY-FREE

6 cups water

3 (2-inch) pieces kombu

⅓ cup white miso

8 ounces silken or firm
   tofu, drained, cut
   into small cubes

4 scallions, chopped

1. Combine the water and kombu in a large pot over medium heat. Remove the kombu just as the water starts to come to a boil. Then turn down to a simmer.

2. Place the miso in a small bowl. Scoop out about ½ cup of the broth and pour it over the miso. Whisk together until the miso has dissolved in the water and no lumps remain. Add the miso to the simmering broth. Stir to combine.

3. Reduce the heat to low and add the tofu to the miso broth. Heat through just enough to warm the tofu, 1 to 2 minutes.

4. Just before serving, stir in the scallions.

Ingredient tip: Kombu is dried seaweed, most often used in soups and broths to add an umami flavor.

Flavor boost: For extra depth of flavor, add bonito (dried fish flakes), commonly found in Asian markets.

Storage tip: Store miso soup in the refrigerator for 3 to 4 days.

Per serving: Calories: 60; Fat: 2g; Protein: 3g; Cholesterol: 0mg; Sodium: 610mg; Carbohydrates: 4g; Fiber: 3g

Dashi

SERVES 6 | PREP TIME 5 MINUTES | **COOK TIME** 10 MINUTES

Japanese dashi is a very simple broth made from kombu and dried bonito flakes. The kombu and bonito are rich with umami and give this simple soup an extra layer of savory flavor and complexity.

FAST, FREEZER
FRIENDLY, DAIRY-FREE
GLUTEN-FREE,
QUICK PREP

6 cups water

3 (2-inch) pieces kombu

1 cup dried bonito flakes

1. Combine the water and kombu in a large pot over medium heat. Remove the kombu just as the water starts to come to a boil. (Boiling the kombu can make the broth bitter and a bit slimy.)

2. Turn broth down to a simmer. Add the bonito flakes and simmer for 1 minute. Remove the pot from the heat and let the bonito flakes steep in the broth for 5 minutes.

3. Strain the bonito flakes from the broth using a fine-mesh strainer.

Storage tip: This broth can be used immediately, refrigerated for up to a week, or frozen for up to 3 months.

Storage tip: Have leftover kombu and bonito flakes? Store in the freezer for up to a year in an airtight container.

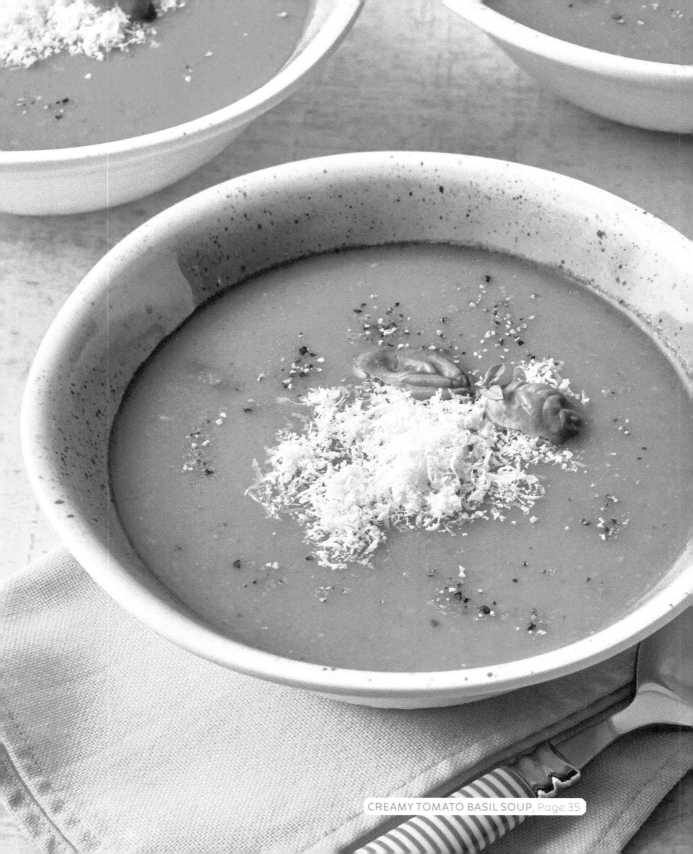

CREAMY TOMATO BASIL SOUP, Page 35

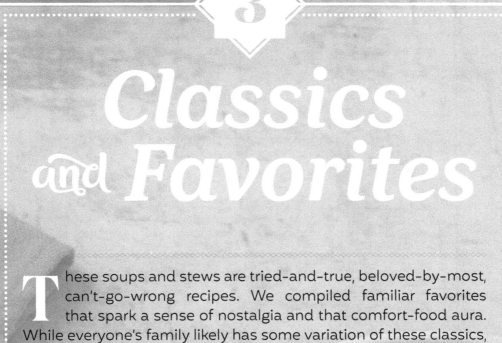

3

Classics and Favorites

These soups and stews are tried-and-true, beloved-by-most, can't-go-wrong recipes. We compiled familiar favorites that spark a sense of nostalgia and that comfort-food aura. While everyone's family likely has some variation of these classics, we made some subtle changes to enhance their nutritional value and healing properties. Look to this chapter for the most traditional version, then discover spin-off recipes in later chapters. Enjoy!

Classic Chicken Noodle Soup

SERVES 8 | **PREP TIME** 15 MINUTES | **COOK TIME** 30 MINUTES

This soul-warming soup instantly evokes comfort and healing. It may trigger memories of being served chicken noodle soup by a loved one when you were feeling sick. You may even swear that you're feeling better immediately after that first sip. The onions, carrots, and celery contain vitamins A and C and other antioxidants that have been known to build a strong immune system and fight off viruses. They may help the body recover from illness more quickly.

DAIRY-FREE

3 tablespoons olive oil

1 large onion, chopped

3 large carrots, peeled and chopped

4 celery stalks, chopped

4 garlic cloves, minced

10 cups Chicken Broth (page 24)

8 ounces egg noodles

4 cups shredded cooked chicken breast

Salt

Black pepper

½ cup fresh parsley leaves, chopped

1. In a large stockpot, heat the olive oil over medium-high heat. Add the onions, carrots, and celery, stirring frequently until the vegetables are tender, about 15 minutes.

2. Add the garlic and cook for an additional 1 minute or until fragrant. Add the broth and bring to a boil.

3. Add the egg noodles and cook for 6 minutes. Then add the shredded chicken and cook for an additional 2 minutes, until the noodles are cooked through and the chicken has warmed.

4. Season with salt and pepper to taste. Stir in the parsley.

Substitution tip: To make this gluten-free, simply use a gluten-free noodle variety. The cooking time may change depending on the noodle type.

Ingredient tip: Save time by using a store-bought rotisserie chicken. Simply shred the breast meat. Then, save the bones in your freezer to create a nourishing chicken stock (see page 25).

Flavor boost: Looking for a kick of heat? Toss the shredded chicken with 1 teaspoon of chili powder before adding to the soup.

Per serving: Calories: 320; Fat: 9g; Protein: 31g; Cholesterol: 85mg; Sodium: 210mg; Carbohydrates: 27g; Fiber: 3g

Creamy Tomato Basil Soup

SERVES 8 | PREP TIME 10 MINUTES | **COOK TIME** 40 MINUTES

There's really nothing more comforting than a steaming hot bowl of tomato soup. We prefer using canned tomatoes rather than fresh, not only for convenience, but because they are packed in peak season—that means they're perfectly ripe! Canned tomatoes are loaded with powerful antioxidants, such as beta-carotene and lycopene. Lycopene has been found to be more absorbable by the body in its cooked form, and because tomatoes are cooked during the canning process, they actually have more of the lycopene than the raw variety.

FREEZER FRIENDLY,
QUICK PREP

2 tablespoons olive oil

1 large Vidalia onion,
  chopped

3 garlic cloves, minced

2 tablespoons all-
  purpose flour

3 cups Chicken Broth
  (page 24)

1 (28-ounce) can whole
  peeled tomatoes,
  with juices

1 teaspoon sugar

¼ cup chopped fresh basil

1 cup whole milk

Salt

Black pepper

Shredded Parmesan
  cheese (optional)

1. In a large pot, heat the olive oil over medium-high heat. Add the onion and sauté until translucent, 5 to 7 minutes. Then add the garlic and cook until fragrant, 1 to 2 minutes.

2. Add the flour and stir to coat the onion and garlic.

3. Add the broth and tomatoes with their juices. Bring to a simmer, while stirring to make sure all the ingredients are incorporated and the flour is not sticking to the bottom of the pan. Reduce the heat to low, cover, and simmer for 30 minutes.

4. Turn off the heat. Stir in the sugar, basil, and milk to combine.

5. Using an immersion blender, blend the soup until creamy. Alternatively, in small batches using a high-speed blender, blend the soup until smooth.

6. Season with salt and pepper to taste. Top with Parmesan cheese, if using.

Flavor boost: An important factor in achieving great tomato flavor is balancing acidity and sweetness. Too much of either can leave you with a tomato sauce that tastes one-dimensional. To balance the tomato acidity, add a bit of sugar.

Continued

Creamy Tomato Basil Soup *Continued*

Flavor boost: When your soup is simmering, throw in a rind of Parmesan cheese. The rind will soften, and the flavors of the cheese will infuse the dish. Remove any undissolved rind when you're ready to blend the soup.

Per serving: Calories: 210; Fat: 12g; Protein: 7g; Cholesterol: 5mg; Sodium: 380mg; Carbohydrates: 20g; Fiber: 3g

Egg Drop Soup

SERVES 8 | **PREP TIME** 10 MINUTES | **COOK TIME** 20 MINUTES

This popular Chinese restaurant menu staple is made from a flavorful broth filled with delicious egg "ribbons," which are created by whisking raw eggs into the simmering broth. Eggs are an all-natural source of high-quality protein and a number of other nutrients, all for 70 calories per large egg.

DAIRY-FREE, FAST,
QUICK PREP

8 cups Chicken Stock
   (page 25)

1 tablespoon finely
   grated fresh ginger

1 tablespoon low-
   sodium soy sauce

1½ tablespoons cornstarch

3 large eggs

1 tablespoon toasted
   sesame oil

Salt

White pepper or
   black pepper

4 scallions, thinly sliced

1. In a large pot, bring the stock and ginger to a boil.

2. In a small bowl, whisk together the soy sauce and cornstarch until the cornstarch has dissolved. If more liquid is needed to dissolve the cornstarch, use a little of the broth. Add the soy sauce mixture to the stock and boil for an additional 1 to 2 minutes, until the soup has slightly thickened. Remove the pot from the heat.

3. In a medium bowl, whisk together the eggs, sesame oil, and salt and pepper to taste. Slowly pour the egg mixture into the hot broth, whisking constantly to break up the eggs as they cook in the soup.

4. Season with additional salt and pepper. Garnish with the scallions.

Substitution tip: To make this gluten-free, use a gluten-free soy sauce, like tamari.

Ingredient tip: Traditionally, this soup is made with white pepper, which has a different flavor than black pepper. It also tends to be stronger, so if you choose to use white pepper in this recipe, start with a conservative amount and adjust according to your taste preference.

Per serving: Calories: 140; Fat: 6g; Protein: 9g; Cholesterol: 75mg; Sodium: 460mg; Carbohydrates: 11g; Fiber: 0g

Italian Wedding Soup

SERVES 10 | PREP TIME 30 MINUTES | **COOK TIME** 30 MINUTES

The term "wedding soup" comes from the Italian phrase "minestra maritata" ("married soup"), which refers to the combination or "marriage" of greens and meat. Traditionally, acini di pepe pasta is used. It looks like little pearls. If you are unable to find that at the grocery store, use ditalini or orzo pasta instead. Filled with home-made meatballs, fresh veggies, and bits of pasta, this is a bowl of goodness to be served any time during the year.

For the meatballs

1 pound 93% lean ground turkey

½ cup whole-wheat bread crumbs

1 egg, beaten

2 tablespoons grated Parmesan cheese

1 tablespoon garlic powder

½ tablespoon fennel seeds

1 tablespoon Italian seasoning

½ teaspoon salt

¼ teaspoon black pepper

For the soup

1 tablespoon olive oil

1 small onion, chopped

2 large carrots, peeled and chopped

2 celery stalks, chopped

4 garlic cloves, minced

To make the meatballs

1. Preheat the oven to 400°F. Line a baking sheet with parchment paper.

2. In a large bowl, combine the turkey, bread crumbs, egg, Parmesan cheese, garlic powder, fennel seeds, Italian seasoning, salt, and pepper. Mix well to combine.

3. Shape ½-inch meatballs and place on the baking sheet. Bake for 15 to 20 minutes, until the internal temperature reaches 165°F. Remove from the oven and set aside.

8 cups Chicken Stock
(page 25)

2 cups water

½ cup acini di pepe pasta

4 cups baby spinach

Salt

Pepper

½ cup grated Parmesan
cheese (optional)

To make the soup

1. In a large pot, heat the olive oil over medium-high heat. Add the onions, carrots, and celery and cook for 5 to 7 minutes, until the onions are translucent and the vegetables are tender. Add the garlic and cook for an additional 2 minutes.

2. Add the stock, water, and pasta. Bring to a boil then reduce to a simmer for 10 to 15 minutes, until the pasta is tender. Add the meatballs and spinach and cook until the meatballs are warmed through and the spinach has wilted, 3 to 5 minutes.

3. Season with salt and pepper to taste. Top with Parmesan cheese, if using.

Freezer-friendly tip: Make a double batch of the meatballs and freeze half to use later.

Flavor boost: Traditional Italian wedding soup is often made with a mixture of beef and sausage for the meatballs. Using ground turkey is a leaner option. The addition of the fennel seeds adds a familiar sausage taste.

Substitution tip: Kale, endive, and escarole are other greens commonly used in Italian wedding soup, and they would work well in this recipe.

Per serving: Calories: 220; Fat: 8g; Protein: 13g; Cholesterol: 40mg; Sodium: 560mg; Carbohydrates: 25g; Fiber: 2g

Minestrone Soup

SERVES 8 | **PREP TIME** 20 MINUTES | **COOK TIME** 40 MINUTES

This super easy minestrone soup is a one-pot meal that is full of vegetables, pasta, and an incredible tomato base. It makes a satisfying dinner for a cool fall day! It's quick, it's healthy, and it's perfect for dunking with some crusty bread or rolls!

VEGETARIAN

2 tablespoons olive oil

1 large onion, diced

5 garlic cloves, minced

3 celery stalks, diced

2 large carrots, peeled and diced

½ pound green beans, trimmed and cut into ½-inch pieces

1 teaspoon dried oregano

1 teaspoon dried basil

1 teaspoon dried parsley

1 (28-ounce) can no-salt-added diced tomatoes

1 (14-ounce) can no-salt-added crushed tomatoes

1. In a large pot, heat the oil over medium-high heat. Add the onion and cook until translucent, about 3 minutes. Add the garlic and cook for 1 minute or until fragrant.

2. Add the celery and carrots, stir to combine, and cook until they begin to soften, about 5 minutes.

3. Stir in the green beans, oregano, basil, and parsley, cooking for 3 minutes.

4. Add the diced and crushed tomatoes and broth to the pot. Bring to a boil, then reduce to a simmer for 10 minutes.

5. Stir in the kidney beans and pasta and simmer for an additional 10 minutes, until the pasta and vegetables are tender.

6. Season with salt and pepper to taste. Top with Parmesan cheese, if desired.

8 cups Classic Vegetable
  Broth (page 22)

1 (15-ounce) can dark
  red kidney beans,
  drained and rinsed

1 cup conchiglie pasta
  (small shells)

Salt

Black pepper

Grated Parmesan
  cheese (optional)

Flavor boost: When your soup is simmering, throw in a Parmesan rind. If the rind hasn't completely dissolved by the time you're ready to serve, remove the remaining rind.

Substitution tip: Any small pasta will work for this recipe, like elbow or ditalini. If using whole-wheat or bean-based pasta, you may need to adjust with additional water or broth, as they tend to absorb more liquid.

Substitution tip: Minestrone was traditionally made to use up leftover vegetables, so feel free to use any vegetables and greens you have on hand.

Per serving: Calories: 210; Fat: 4.5g; Protein: 7g; Cholesterol: 0mg; Sodium: 640mg; Carbohydrates: 36g; Fiber: 8g

Matzo Ball Soup

SERVES 8 | PREP TIME 15 MINUTES, 2 HOURS TO CHILL | **COOK TIME** 45 MINUTES

When Julie worked as a private chef, she cooked for a Jewish family and learned their family secrets to create delicious and tender matzo balls. Matzo ball soup is traditionally enjoyed during Passover, a time when leavened foods are restricted. Using club soda in the matzo mix physically creates gas bubbles mimicking the leavening process. The other key ingredient to matzo balls is schmaltz, or rendered chicken fat. It gives the matzo balls most of their flavor. Look for frozen rendered chicken fat in the kosher section of your grocery store, or ask a local butcher.

DAIRY-FREE

1 cup matzo meal

3 large eggs, lightly beaten

3 tablespoons chicken fat

1 teaspoon salt

½ tablespoon chopped
    fresh parsley

¼ cup club soda

½ cup boiling water

10 cups Chicken
    Stock (page 25)

1. In a large bowl, mix together the matzo meal, eggs, chicken fat, salt, and parsley. Pour in the club soda and stir to combine. Then pour in the boiling water and let sit until the water is mostly absorbed and no dry crumbs remain. The mixture will resemble wet sand. Cover and refrigerate for at least 2 hours.

2. Heat the stock in a large stockpot to a simmer.

3. Using wet hands, gently form rounded tablespoons of the matzo ball mixture into 1-inch balls, transferring to a parchment-lined plate. (Do not overwork the mixture, or it will become too dense.)

4. Add the matzo balls to the stock and return to a gentle simmer. Turn the heat down to low, cover, and simmer for 40 to 45 minutes, until matzo balls have doubled in size and are cooked through (meaning no raw dough in the center).

5. Ladle into bowls and garnish with additional parsley, if desired.

Substitution tip: Can't find schmaltz? You can substitute oil or butter (though butter conflicts with kosher dietary restrictions prohibiting combining meat with dairy).

Flavor boost: Add other aromatics—like onions, garlic, carrots, celery—and cooked shredded chicken to the broth with matzo balls.

Per serving: Calories: 230; Fat: 10g; Protein: 11g; Cholesterol: 85mg; Sodium: 750mg; Carbohydrates: 22g; Fiber: 0g

Potato Cauliflower Leek Soup

SERVES 6 | PREP TIME 15 MINUTES | **COOK TIME** 30 MINUTES

This is a French cuisine classic, but we added immune-boosting cauliflower for a nutritious base. To save a few minutes of chopping, you can substitute frozen chopped cauliflower for fresh. You can use your favorite dairy milk alternative, including almond, coconut, and oat milk. This recipe can also use soy or cow's milk, if you prefer.

DAIRY-FREE,
FREEZER FRIENDLY,
GLUTEN-FREE, VEGAN

2 tablespoons olive oil

3 leeks, halved lengthwise
   and chopped

4 garlic cloves, minced

2 large russet potatoes,
   peeled and cut into
   a small dice

2 cauliflower heads, cut into
   small florets (about 5 cups)

5 cups Classic Vegetable
   Broth (page 22)

3 thyme sprigs

2 bay leaves

1 cup nondairy milk of choice

Salt

Black pepper

2 tablespoons chopped
   chives for garnish

1. In a large pot, heat the olive oil over medium-high heat. Add the leeks and garlic and sauté for 3 minutes.

2. Add the potatoes and cauliflower and stir to combine. Add the broth, thyme, and bay leaves and bring to a boil, making sure all the vegetables are fully submerged in the broth. Then reduce the heat and simmer for 25 minutes, until the cauliflower and potatoes are fork tender. Remove the thyme and bay leaves.

3. Using an immersion blender, purée the soup until creamy. Stir in the nondairy milk. If a thinner soup consistency is desired, add more milk or broth and purée until the desired consistency is reached. Alternatively, add the soup to a high-speed blender in small batches to purée.

4. Season with salt and pepper to taste. Garnish with the chives.

Culinary term: Fork tender is when food is cooked so that it can be cut or pierced easily with a fork.

Ingredient tip: Leeks are a root vegetable and are buried in dirt as they grow, and each of their layers catch some dirt inside as it forms. Be sure to clean them thoroughly by slicing them in half horizontally and rinsing with cold water.

Per serving: Calories: 250; Fat: 6g; Protein: 9g; Cholesterol: 0mg; Sodium: 230mg; Carbohydrates: 43g; Fiber: 7g

Clam Chowder

SERVES 6 | PREP TIME 10 MINUTES | **COOK TIME** 30 MINUTES

Clam chowder always sparks a memory of coming inside during a cold winter and opening up a can of soup with crackers. That simple, one-step meal was convenient, but trust us when we say that this recipe is worth the extra effort for the great flavor you'll enjoy at the end. Look for canned or jarred clams (with juice) in the same section as canned tuna or salmon. If you are peeling your potatoes, complete them before prepping the other ingredients.

GLUTEN-FREE, QUICK PREP, FREEZER FRIENDLY

1 tablespoon canola oil

1 large sweet or yellow onion, diced

1 large carrot, peeled and chopped or sliced into thin half-moons

3 celery stalks, cut into ¼-inch slices

2 rosemary sprigs (or 1 tablespoon dried), plus additional for garnish

2 bay leaves

1 cup dry white wine

4 cups Classic Vegetable Broth (page 22)

1. Heat a large Dutch oven or stockpot over medium heat. Add the canola oil and once the oil is glistening, add the onion, carrot, celery, rosemary, and bay leaves. Sauté for 5 to 8 minutes, until the onion becomes translucent and fragrant. Add the wine and stir to deglaze the bottom of the pot.

2. Add the broth and potatoes. Bring to a boil, then reduce the heat and simmer for 15 minutes, until the potatoes become tender. Meanwhile, chop the clams, reserving the juice to add if desired.

3. Carefully ladle half of the soup, liquid included, into a blender. Vent the lid to allow steam to escape, then blend until smooth. Add the purée back to the Dutch oven, along with clam juice, if using, and stir to thicken the chowder.

Continued

3 Russet potatoes, peeled
    if desired and cut
    into ½-inch cubes

2 (6-ounce) cans
    clams, with juice

1 cup frozen or canned
    sweet corn kernels

1 cup whole milk

Salt

Black pepper

4. Add the clams, corn, and milk. Simmer for 5 minutes more, then season with salt and pepper to taste. Serve immediately and garnish with additional rosemary if desired.

Substitution tip: You can replace the white wine with additional vegetable broth to deglaze your pot. Feel free to use other types of seafood in place of or in addition to clams to create a seafood chowder.

Per serving: Calories: 360; Fat: 5g; Protein: 20g; Cholesterol: 30mg; Sodium: 240mg; Carbohydrates: 51g; Fiber: 8g

French Onion Soup

SERVES 8 | PREP TIME 10 MINUTES | **COOK TIME** 2 HOURS 5 MINUTES

A diner staple, French onion soup has sweet caramelized onions and a rich beefy broth that is loved by most everyone!

For the soup

2 tablespoons olive oil

1 tablespoon unsalted butter

3 pounds onions,
    thinly sliced

4 garlic cloves, minced

5 cups Beef Stock (page 26)

Salt

Black pepper

**For optional bread
and cheese topping**

8 baguette slices

1 tablespoon olive oil

2 garlic cloves, halved

¾ cup shredded
    Gruyère cheese

To make the soup

1. In a Dutch oven (or a heavy-bottom pot), heat the olive oil and butter over medium-high heat. Add the onions, cooking and stirring until softened, about 10 minutes. Reduce the heat to medium-low; cover and cook, stirring occasionally, until the onions are deep golden brown, 30 to 40 minutes. Add the garlic; cook 2 minutes longer.

2. Add the stock and stir to combine. Bring to a boil and reduce to a simmer. Cook, covered and occasionally stirring, for 1 hour. Season with salt and pepper to taste.

To make the optional bread and cheese topping

1. Preheat the oven to 400°F. Brush the baguette slices with the olive oil on both sides and place on a baking sheet. Bake for 5 to 7 minutes, flipping halfway through, until toasted and golden brown.

2. Rub the warm bread slices with the flesh of the garlic cloves. Ladle the soup into oven-safe bowls and place on a baking sheet. Place the toast on top of the soup, then add a layer of cheese. Broil for 3 to 5 minutes until the cheese has melted.

Continued

French Onion Soup *Continued*

Ingredient tip: If you want a hint of sweetness, use Vidalia (sweet) onions. Not as confident with your knife skills? Try using a mandoline to slice the onions thin.

Flavor boost: Slowly cooking onions brings out their deep, rich, sweet flavor as the natural sugars in the onions caramelize.

Per serving: Calories: 120; Fat: 1.5g; Protein: 5g; Cholesterol: <5mg; Sodium: 320mg; Carbohydrates: 18g; Fiber: 3g

Per serving (with cheese and bread topping): Calories: 280; Fat: 11g; Protein: 12g; Cholesterol: 15mg; Sodium: 560mg; Carbohydrates: 37g; Fiber: 4g

Split Pea Soup

SERVES 6 | PREP TIME 20 MINUTES | **COOK TIME** 2 HOURS

Traditionally, split pea soup is made by simmering a ham hock. Our vegan twist results in a smoky and flavorful soup utilizing anti-inflammatory herbs and spices, like garam masala, an Indian spice blend. Garam masala traditionally consists of coriander, cumin, cardamom, cloves, black pepper, and nutmeg. If you don't have this blend on hand, make your own (see the substitution tip).

FREEZER FRIENDLY,
GLUTEN-FREE, VEGAN,
DAIRY-FREE

2 tablespoons olive oil

2 medium onions, chopped

2 carrots, peeled
   and chopped

3 celery stalks, chopped

2 cups green split peas

½ teaspoon dried basil

1 teaspoon ground cumin

½ teaspoon garam masala

2 bay leaves

6 cups Classic Vegetable
   Broth (page 22)

1 cup water

Salt

Black pepper

1. In a large pot, heat the olive oil over medium-high heat. Add the onions, carrots, and celery. Sauté until the onions are translucent and the vegetables are tender, 5 to 7 minutes.

2. Stir in the split peas, basil, cumin, garam masala, and bay leaves.

3. Add the broth and stir to combine. Bring to a boil, then reduce to a low simmer. Cover and cook for 1½ hours, stirring every 30 minutes, until the peas are tender.

4. Stir and adjust the consistency by adding ½ cup of water at a time.

5. Remove the bay leaves. Season with salt and pepper to taste.

Substitution tip: No garam masala? Create your own spice blend with a combination of 1 tablespoon ground cumin, 1½ teaspoons ground coriander, 1½ teaspoons ground cardamom, 1½ teaspoons black pepper, 1 teaspoon cinnamon, ½ teaspoon ground cloves, and ½ teaspoon ground nutmeg. Place the mix in an airtight container, and store in a cool, dry place.

Per serving: Calories: 230; Fat: 4.5g; Protein: 16g; Cholesterol: 0mg; Sodium: 240mg; Carbohydrates: 45g; Fiber: 18g

Broccoli Cheddar Soup

SERVES 6 | PREP TIME 5 MINUTES | **COOK TIME** 35 MINUTES

Broccoli cheddar soup is one of the most popular soup recipes in existence. It graces nearly every restaurant menu and has spawned countless variations. This version goes back to basics and keeps things simple—and quick! You can have a welcoming bowl in less than 40 minutes.

FAST, FREEZER FRIENDLY, QUICK PREP, VEGETARIAN

1/3 cup olive oil

1 large yellow onion, chopped

3 garlic cloves, minced

1/3 cup all-purpose flour

3 cups Classic Vegetable Broth (page 22)

2 cups whole milk

Salt

Black pepper

1 teaspoon mustard powder

1/8 teaspoon allspice

1/8 teaspoon nutmeg

4 cups finely chopped broccoli florets

2 large carrots, peeled and grated

2 cups shredded sharp cheddar cheese

1. Heat the olive oil in a large stockpot or Dutch oven over medium heat. Add the onion and cook until translucent, about 2 minutes. Add the garlic and cook 1 minute more. Whisk in the flour and create a simple roux. Allow to cook until golden brown, 2 to 3 minutes.

2. Reduce the heat to medium-low and add the broth and milk, whisking to dissolve the roux into the liquid. Season with salt and pepper, then add the mustard powder, allspice, and nutmeg.

3. Add the broccoli and carrots and gently simmer for 15 to 20 minutes, until the broccoli is tender. Add the cheese, reserving a small amount for topping. Transfer to serving bowls, garnish with the reserved cheese, and serve immediately.

Ingredient tip: This recipe is quite filling as it is, but if you prefer some additional protein, try adding chickpeas or shredded or chopped chicken. You can also add more vegetables if desired.

Culinary term: Roux is used as a thickening agent for gravy, sauces, soups, and stews. It is made from equal parts flour and fat cooked together. Commonly used fats include butter, vegetable oils, or bacon drippings.

Per serving: Calories: 390; Fat: 27g; Protein: 13g; Cholesterol: 50mg; Sodium: 400mg; Carbohydrates: 20g; Fiber: 3g

Simple Homemade Ramen

SERVES 6 | **PREP TIME** 10 MINUTES | **COOK TIME** 20 MINUTES

Skip the sodium bomb instant version and make a fresh and flavorful batch of home-made ramen. Authentic ramen usually takes hours to cook to develop. We added a few flavor-boosting ingredients like garlic, ginger, and soy sauce, which help create bold flavors in a shorter amount of time. This is also great with mushroom broth (see page 29) or a vegetable broth (see pages 22 and 23) for a vegetarian version.

QUICK PREP, FAST,
DAIRY-FREE

1 tablespoon sesame oil

3 teaspoons grated
fresh ginger

3 garlic cloves, minced

1 cup shredded carrots

8 ounces shiitake
mushrooms, *thinly sliced*

4 cups Chicken Broth
(page 24)

4 cups water

2 tablespoons low-
sodium soy sauce

2 packages instant ramen
(noodles only; discard
seasoning packet)

Salt

Black pepper

Sliced scallions, sesame
seeds, sriracha sauce,
and soft-boiled egg, for
topping (optional)

1. In a large pot, heat the sesame oil over medium-high heat. Add the ginger and garlic, and cook until fragrant, about 1 minute.

2. Add the carrots and mushrooms; sauté for an additional 2 minutes, until they begin to soften.

3. Add the broth, water, and soy sauce. Bring to a boil, then reduce to a simmer. Let simmer for 5 minutes.

4. Place the ramen noodles in the simmering broth, stirring to combine, and cook for about 3 minutes until noodles are tender.

5. Season with salt and pepper. Add toppings, if using.

Substitution tip: Use cremini mushrooms (also known as baby portobellos) if they are easier to find.

Ingredient tip: To make a soft-boiled egg, bring water to a boil in a small saucepan. Add the egg, and let it boil for 6 minutes. Remove the egg and submerge into an ice bath for a minute to cool it off enough to handle. Lightly crack and roll the egg on a flat surface, peel, slice in half, and place on top of your ramen.

Per serving: Calories: 170; Fat: 3.5g; Protein: 9g; Cholesterol: 0mg; Sodium: 510mg; Carbohydrates: 28g; Fiber: 3g

Chicken and Wild Rice Soup

SERVES 6 | PREP TIME 10 MINUTES | **COOK TIME** 1 HOUR

The stovetop version of this soup is worth the wait: It's thick and creamy but doesn't rely on heavy cream or thickeners. The trick? Using an immersion blender to take advantage of the natural starches in rice and potatoes. When combined with milk, they create a much creamier texture than if left unblended.

FREEZER FRIENDLY,
QUICK PREP,
GLUTEN-FREE

2 tablespoons olive oil

1 large yellow onion, diced

3 garlic cloves, minced

2 large carrots, peeled
   and chopped

2 large celery stalks, diced

8 ounces baby bella or
   white mushrooms, sliced

1 pound boneless, skinless
   chicken breasts

2 large potatoes, peeled
   if desired and cut
   into ½-inch cubes

1 cup wild rice

8 cups Chicken Broth
   (page 24)

2 teaspoons dried
   thyme, divided

Salt

Pepper

2 cups whole milk

1 tablespoon Dijon mustard

1 teaspoon garlic powder

Chopped fresh parsley,
   for garnish

1. Heat the olive oil in a large stockpot or Dutch oven over medium heat. Add the onion, garlic, carrots, celery, and mushrooms. Sauté for 5 minutes, then add the chicken, potatoes, wild rice, broth, 1 teaspoon thyme, salt, and pepper.

2. Bring to a boil, then reduce the heat and simmer with the lid vented for about 45 minutes.

3. Once the chicken is fully cooked (to 165°F), transfer to a plate and shred with two forks. With chicken still removed, add the milk, mustard, 1 teaspoon thyme, and garlic powder. Use an immersion blender to pulse a few times. Continue to your desired thickness, leaving some larger chunks of vegetables and potatoes. Return the chicken to the pot and stir to combine.

4. Season with salt and pepper to taste. Garnish with parsley and serve immediately.

To use a slow cooker: Add all ingredients except the milk, mustard, thyme, and garlic powder to the bowl of your slow cooker. Cook on high for 5 to 6 hours or low for 8 to 10 hours. Follow steps 3 and 4 as written.

Per serving: Calories: 460; Fat: 12g; Protein: 35g; Cholesterol: 65mg; Sodium: 300mg; Carbohydrates: 57g; Fiber: 5g

Cream of Mushroom

SERVES 6 | **PREP TIME** 10 MINUTES | **COOK TIME** 35 MINUTES

The deep, earthy flavors of a homemade cream of mushroom soup can't be beat, especially when it's ready in minutes. You'll never open a can of mushroom soup after trying our recipe!

QUICK PREP, FREEZER FRIENDLY

3 tablespoons unsalted butter

1 tablespoon canola oil

1 large onion, diced

1½ pounds cremini mushrooms, sliced

4 garlic cloves, minced

2 teaspoons dried thyme

½ cup dry red wine (like marsala)

6 tablespoons all-purpose flour

4 cups Chicken Stock (page 25), divided

Salt

Black pepper

1 cup heavy cream

Chopped fresh parsley, for garnish

1. In a large pot, heat the butter and canola oil over medium-high heat. Add the onions and mushrooms and sauté until tender, about 5 to 7 minutes. Add the garlic and thyme and sauté until fragrant, 1 to 2 minutes.

2. Add the wine and cook until reduced by half.

3. In a small bowl, whisk in the flour with 2 cups of stock. Add to the pot with the remaining 2 cups of stock, salt, and pepper. Bring to a boil, then reduce to a simmer. Cover and allow to simmer for 10 to 15 minutes, occasionally stirring, until thickened.

4. Reduce the heat, stir in the cream, and cook until the flavors have blended. Season with salt and pepper to taste. Garnish with parsley.

Flavor boost: Cremini mushrooms have a deeper, earthier flavor than white button mushrooms. Creminis' hearty taste makes them an excellent addition to beef, wild game, and vegetable dishes.

Flavor boost: As a cooking ingredient, wine imparts its flavors, body, acidity, and even some of its subtleties.

Per serving: Calories: 350; Fat: 25g; Protein: 9g; Cholesterol: 75mg; Sodium: 280mg; Carbohydrates: 21g; Fiber: 1g

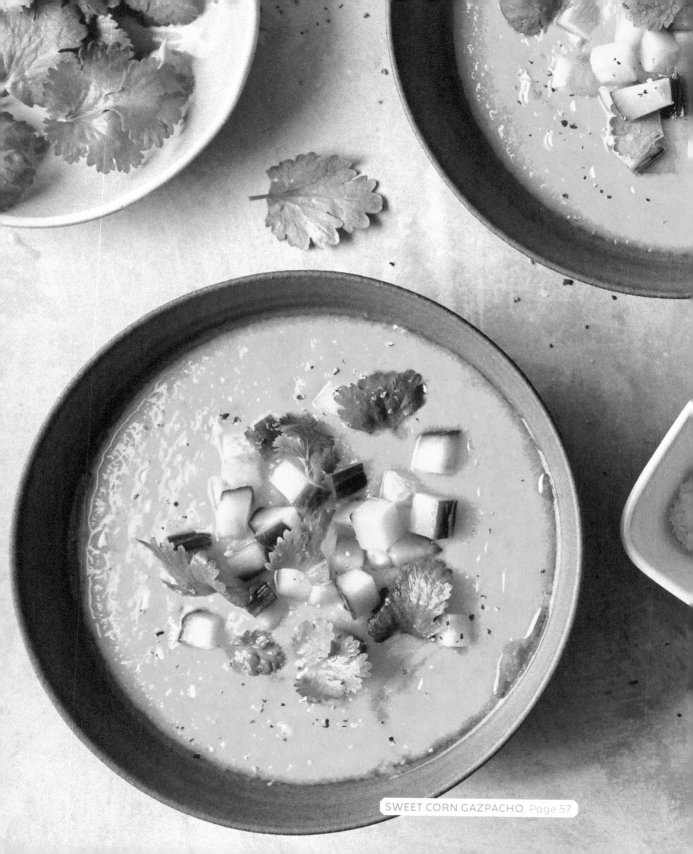

SWEET CORN GAZPACHO, Page 57

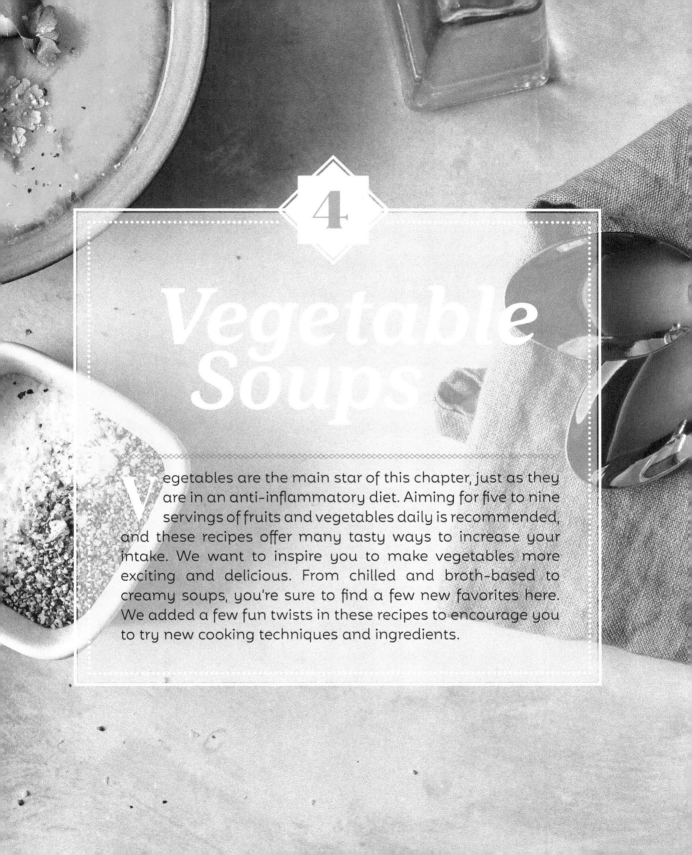

4

Vegetable Soups

Vegetables are the main star of this chapter, just as they are in an anti-inflammatory diet. Aiming for five to nine servings of fruits and vegetables daily is recommended, and these recipes offer many tasty ways to increase your intake. We want to inspire you to make vegetables more exciting and delicious. From chilled and broth-based to creamy soups, you're sure to find a few new favorites here. We added a few fun twists in these recipes to encourage you to try new cooking techniques and ingredients.

Gazpacho

SERVES 4 | PREP TIME 20 MINUTES, 2 HOURS TO CHILL

A classic of Spanish cuisine, gazpacho originated in the southern region of Andalusia. It is the quintessential summer soup not only because it's served chilled but also because all of the seasonal ingredients are at the peak of ripeness.

GLUTEN-FREE,
DAIRY-FREE, VEGAN

2 large beefsteak tomatoes

1 English cucumber

1 medium red onion

1 (15-ounce) jar roasted
    red peppers, drained

3 cups low-sodium
    tomato juice

1 cilantro bunch, chopped
    (about ½ cup)

⅓ cup red wine vinegar

¼ cup olive oil

Hot sauce

Salt

Black pepper

1. Chop one tomato, half the cucumber, and half the onion into 1-inch pieces. Transfer to a blender with the roasted red peppers, tomato juice, cilantro, vinegar, olive oil, and hot sauce. Purée until smooth. Transfer to a bowl and set aside.

2. Seed the remaining tomato and chop into a small dice, as well as the remaining cucumber and red onion. Stir into the soup.

3. Season with salt and pepper to taste. Refrigerate at least 2 hours before serving. Serve chilled.

Ingredient tip: English cucumbers, also known as seedless cucumbers, are found wrapped in plastic at the grocery store. Why? Because they have a more delicate skin. If you are not using an English cucumber, then simply scoop out the seeds of the conventional cucumber, which tend to be bitter.

Storage tip: This recipe can be made up to 2 days in advance. As it sits in the refrigerator, the flavors will deepen.

Per serving: Calories: 190; Fat: 0g; Protein: 7g; Cholesterol: 0mg; Sodium: 220mg; Carbohydrates: 41g; Fiber: 7g

Sweet Corn Gazpacho

SERVES 4 | PREP TIME 5 MINUTES, 25 MINUTES TO CHILL

This simple soup is another take on gazpacho, but it uses sweet corn kernels as a base. You can substitute any variety of sweet cherry tomatoes you are able to find or use a red bell pepper instead of yellow; just be prepared for the color to vary depending on the ingredients you use! Note that the consistency of this version will be thicker than a traditional gazpacho, but you can adjust by adding tomato juice.

DAIRY-FREE, FAST, GLUTEN-FREE, QUICK PREP, VEGAN

1½ cups sweet corn kernels

3 cups halved sungold tomatoes

1 large yellow or orange bell pepper, diced (about 1½ cups)

½ cup diced onion

¼ cup olive oil

1½ tablespoons white balsamic vinegar

Salt

Black pepper

1 cup diced cucumber, for garnish

Fresh cilantro, for garnish

1. Combine the corn, tomatoes, bell pepper, and onion in a large mixing bowl. Transfer to a high-speed blender and blend until completely smooth or blend in batches if needed to achieve a smooth consistency. Let soup chill for 25 minutes.

2. Pour into serving bowls and drizzle with the olive oil and vinegar. Season with salt and pepper to taste. Top each serving with diced cucumber and garnish with fresh cilantro.

Ingredient tip: Make the most of summer sweet corn by using fresh kernels instead of frozen or canned. To safely and efficiently remove corn kernels from the cob, blanch the corn ears or steam them in the microwave. Use a chef's knife to cut off the narrow tip of the ear, giving you a flat surface to place in the center of a plate. Grip the top of the ear of corn by the stem, then use your knife to cut vertically down, separating the kernels from the cob. Rotate the cob and repeat until the ear is stripped and you have a sufficient amount of corn.

Ingredient tip: Dark balsamic vinegar is slightly sweeter and tends to be more syrupy than white balsamic vinegar, which has a cleaner aftertaste that is ideal for this light recipe.

Per serving: Calories: 210; Fat: 14g; Protein: 4g; Cholesterol: 0mg; Sodium: 50mg; Carbohydrates: 22g; Fiber: 3g

Miso, Ginger, Mushroom Soup

SERVES 8 | PREP TIME 10 MINUTES **| COOK TIME** 20 MINUTES

Similar to the miso soup (see page 30), this version adds notes of pungent ginger and savory mushrooms. Ready in about 30 minutes, this nourishing brothy soup can be served as a starter to any meal.

DAIRY-FREE, QUICK
PREP, FAST

8 cups Dashi (page 31) or
  Mushroom Broth (page 29)

8 ounces cremini
  mushrooms, thinly sliced

2 tablespoons grated
  fresh ginger

2 garlic cloves, grated

⅓ cup white miso

2 tablespoons low-
  sodium soy sauce

6 ounces soft tofu, drained
  and cut in small cubes

Salt

Black pepper

4 scallions, sliced

1. Bring the dashi to a boil in a large saucepan over medium-high heat. Add the mushrooms, ginger, and garlic. Reduce to a simmer and cook for 5 minutes, until mushrooms are tender.

2. In a small bowl, whisk together the miso and soy sauce. Whisk the miso and soy sauce mixture into the broth.

3. Add the tofu and cook for an additional 1 to 2 minutes, until the tofu is warmed through.

4. Season with salt and pepper to taste. Ladle the soup into bowls and top with the scallions.

Ingredient tip: To grate ginger and garlic, use a Microplane. The flavor will infuse into the broth.

Ingredient tip: Tofu is a good source of protein and contains all nine essential amino acids. It is also a valuable plant source of iron and calcium and the minerals manganese, selenium, and phosphorous. If you prefer more of a bite to your tofu, use firm or extra-firm.

Per serving: Calories: 60; Fat: 1.5g; Protein: 5g; Cholesterol: 0mg; Sodium: 550mg; Carbohydrates: 5g; Fiber: 2g

Hot and Sour Soup

SERVES 6 | **PREP TIME** 5 MINUTES | **COOK TIME** 15 MINUTES

Chinese restaurant–style hot and sour soup made easy! This spicy, sour soup is loaded with mushrooms, silky eggs, and tofu. This soup offers a balance of flavors, both yin and yang. Not only does it cater to your taste buds but consuming hot liquid and inhaling steam can help reduce stuffiness and speed up recovery when you are sick.

FAST, QUICK PREP, DAIRY-FREE

8 cups Chicken Broth (page 24)

8 ounces baby bella mushrooms, *thinly sliced*

4 ounces shiitake mushrooms, *thinly sliced*

¼ cup rice vinegar

2 tablespoons low-sodium soy sauce

2 teaspoons ground ginger

1 teaspoon sriracha or chili garlic sauce

¼ cup cornstarch

3 large eggs

8 ounces firm tofu, *drained and cut into ½-inch cubes*

4 scallions, *thinly sliced, divided*

White pepper or black pepper

1. Set aside ¼ cup of the broth. Add the remaining broth, mushrooms, vinegar, soy sauce, ginger, and sriracha to a large stockpot. Stir to combine and heat over medium-high heat until simmering.

2. While soup is heating, whisk the reserved ¼ cup of broth with the cornstarch to make a smooth slurry. When the soup reaches a simmer, slowly stir in the cornstarch slurry. Bring to a boil to allow to thicken, then reduce the heat back to a simmer.

3. Whisk the eggs together in a measuring cup. Slowly stir the soup in a circular motion, then drizzle the egg mixture into the simmering soup to create ribbons of egg in the liquid. Stir in the tofu, half of the scallions, and season with pepper to taste.

4. Garnish with the remaining scallions and serve immediately.

Ingredient tip: Usually, this soup is made with white pepper, which tends to be stronger than black pepper and has a different flavor. If you use white pepper, start with a conservative amount and adjust according to your taste.

Per serving: Calories: 230; Fat: 9g; Protein: 20g; Cholesterol: 95mg; Sodium: 410mg; Carbohydrates: 20g; Fiber: 2g

Ginger Bok Choy and Poached Egg Soup

SERVES 4 | PREP TIME 10 MINUTES | **COOK TIME** 20 MINUTES

Bok choy is a type of Chinese cabbage and, like many other cabbages and crucifer-ous vegetables, it possesses sulfur-based compounds that may help lower the risk of developing chronic diseases.

DAIRY-FREE, FAST,
QUICK PREP,
VEGETARIAN

1 tablespoon sesame oil

½ inch knob fresh ginger,
peeled and sliced

3 garlic cloves, sliced thinly

6 cups Classic Vegetable
Broth (page 22)

2 tablespoons low-
sodium soy sauce

3 bunches baby bok
choy, ends trimmed,
roughly chopped

4 eggs

Salt

Black pepper

2 scallions, thinly
sliced, for garnish

1. In a large wide pot, heat the sesame oil over medium-high heat. Add the ginger and garlic and cook, stirring constantly, until fragrant and garlic begins to brown, 1 to 2 minutes.

2. Add the broth and soy sauce. Stir to combine. Bring to a boil.

3. Add the bok choy and stir to combine.

4. Lower the heat to maintain a gentle simmer. Gently crack the eggs into the soup, keeping the eggs as far apart from each other as possible. Simmer undis-turbed until the whites are set but the yolks are still runny, 3 to 4 minutes.

5. Season with salt and pepper to taste. Top with the scallions and serve immediately.

Ingredient tip: Baby bok choy has a mild, bitter taste with a slightly sweet but peppery flavor and holds up well in soups. Baby bok choy is more tender, but regular bok choy can be used in this recipe as well.

Substitution tip: Sesame oil pairs well with these Asian-inspired flavors, but you can replace it with olive oil.

Per serving: Calories: 220; Fat: 9g; Protein: 17g; Cholesterol: 185mg; Sodium: 1010mg; Carbohydrates: 21g; Fiber: 8g

Golden Vegetable Soup

SERVES 6 | **PREP TIME** 20 MINUTES | **COOK TIME** 30 MINUTES

This may seem like a typical vegetable soup, but the dark orange color will tell you otherwise. The addition of turmeric gives this soup a boost of flavor and health benefits. While uncovering the anti-inflammation compounds of turmeric curcumin, science also discovered antioxidant properties. Antioxidants help fight free radicals in your body, which can cause damaging oxidative stress to healthy cells.

DAIRY-FREE,
FREEZER FRIENDLY,
GLUTEN-FREE, VEGAN

2 tablespoons olive oil

2 large onions, diced

2 large carrots, peeled
  and diced

3 celery stalks, diced

2 tablespoons grated fresh
  turmeric or 2 teaspoons
  ground turmeric

6 garlic cloves, minced

2 tablespoons minced
  fresh ginger

12 cups Classic Vegetable
  Broth (page 22)

4 cups small
  cauliflower florets

5 cups chopped
  stemmed kale

Salt

Black pepper

1. In a large pot, heat the olive oil over medium-high heat. Add the onions, carrots, and celery and cook until the onions are translucent and the vegetables are tender, 5 to 7 minutes.

2. Add the turmeric, garlic, and ginger. Stir to coat the vegetables.

3. Add the broth and bring to a boil.

4. Reduce to a simmer, add the cauliflower, and cover. Cook for 10 to 15 minutes until the cauliflower is tender.

5. Stir in the kale and cook until wilted.

6. Season with salt and pepper to taste.

Ingredient tip: Fresh turmeric is now regularly available at grocery stores. Turmeric contains curcumin, a substance with powerful anti-inflammatory and antioxidant properties. However, it should be noted that beneficial levels of curcumin are difficult to consume through food alone so reach out to a registered dietitian for guidance if you believe you need more.

Per serving: Calories: 160; Fat: 5g; Protein: 5g; Cholesterol: 0mg; Sodium: 380mg; Carbohydrates: 24g; Fiber: 8g

Sun-Dried Tomato and Kale Vegetable Soup

SERVES 8 | PREP TIME 20 MINUTES | **COOK TIME** 30 MINUTES

The flavors in this hearty soup are reminiscent of summer-inspired recipes, but it's filling enough to satisfy in cooler weather. The sun-dried tomatoes provide a concentrated tomato flavor that is the perfect blend of sweet and savory. The addition of whole-wheat pasta and chickpeas rounds out this soup to make it a complete meal.

VEGAN, DAIRY-FREE

2 tablespoons olive oil

2 medium onions, diced

3 carrots, peeled and diced

4 celery stalks, diced

5 garlic cloves, minced

8 ounces cremini mushrooms, sliced

¾ cup sliced sun-dried tomatoes

8 cups Classic Vegetable Broth (page 22)

4 cups water

½ pound whole-wheat ditalini pasta

3 cups chopped stemmed kale

1 (15-ounce) can chickpeas, drained and rinsed

Salt

Pepper

1. In a large stockpot, heat the olive oil over medium heat. Add the onions, carrots, and celery; sweat, allowing the mirepoix to cook slowly and soften without browning, about 6 to 8 minutes. Stir in the garlic and cook for an additional 1 to 2 minutes until fragrant.

2. Add the mushrooms and tomatoes, stirring to combine and cook for 3 to 5 minutes until flavors begin to come together.

3. Add the broth and water to the pot, stir to combine, bring to a boil, then reduce to a simmer.

4. Add the pasta, and cook for 7 to 9 minutes, until the pasta is al dente.

5. Stir in the kale and chickpeas, and cook until the kale has wilted, 3 to 5 minutes.

6. Season with salt and pepper to taste.

Substitution tip: You may substitute Swiss or rainbow chard if kale is unavailable. Strip the inner ribs from the leafy section, then roughly chop the stems separately from the leaves. Add the hardier stems to the soup earlier than the delicate leafy section, which should be added at the very end of cooking.

Ingredient tip: Sun-dried tomatoes are sold dry-packed or in oil. For this recipe use the dry-packed version as they will be reconstituted within the soup.

Per serving: Calories: 250; Fat: 5g; Protein: 9g; Cholesterol: 0mg; Sodium: 300mg; Carbohydrates: 43g; Fiber: 7g

Spicy Sweet Potato Peanut Soup

SERVES 6 | PREP TIME 15 MINUTES | **COOK TIME** 45 MINUTES

Sweet potatoes are a rich source of beta-carotene and vitamin C, which boosts their anti-inflammatory properties. If you prefer a thinner stew, adjust the amount of broth used, as the peanut butter results in an extremely thick texture.

DAIRY-FREE,
GLUTEN-FREE, VEGAN

2 tablespoons olive oil

1 large yellow onion, diced

1 large carrot, peeled
   and diced

2 large celery stalks, diced

4 garlic cloves, minced

1 tablespoon sweet
   curry powder

½ tablespoon ground cumin

1 teaspoon smoked paprika

1 (14.5-ounce) can diced
   tomatoes, with juices

4 cups Classic Vegetable
   Broth (page 22)

1 large sweet potato,
   peeled and cubed

1 (15-ounce) can
   chickpeas, drained

¼ cup creamy or crunchy
   peanut butter

3 cups chopped kale

Salt

Black pepper

½ cup chopped peanuts,
   for garnish

Fresh cilantro, for garnish

1. Heat the olive oil in a large stockpot or Dutch oven over medium-high heat. Add the onion, carrot, and celery and sauté until the onion is translucent, about 5 minutes.

2. Add the garlic, curry powder, cumin, and paprika and stir to combine. Sauté for 1 minute or until fragrant. Add the tomatoes, broth, sweet potatoes, and chickpeas and bring to a boil. Cook for 6 to 8 minutes, uncovered.

3. Reduce the heat to a simmer, cover, and cook for about 20 minutes until the sweet potatoes are soft and the stew begins to thicken. Add the peanut butter and stir to combine. Add the kale and simmer another 3 to 5 minutes.

4. Remove from the heat and season with salt and pepper to taste. Garnish with the peanuts and cilantro. Serve immediately.

Slow cooker option: Add all ingredients except the peanut butter to the bowl of your slow cooker. Cook on high for 3 to 4 hours or on low for 5 to 6 hours. When finished, stir in the peanut butter and serve with peanuts and cilantro.

Per serving: Calories: 330; Fat: 18g; Protein: 13g; Cholesterol: 0mg; Sodium: 450mg; Carbohydrates: 35g; Fiber: 10g

Mushroom and Wild Rice Soup

SERVES 4 | **PREP TIME** 20 MINUTES | **COOK TIME** 2 HOURS 30 MINUTES

Perfectly cozy and comforting, this soup takes a little longer to cook, but it is worth the wait. With savory umami mushrooms paired with the nutty wild rice, you'll be grabbing yourself a second helping.

VEGETARIAN

2 tablespoons olive oil

1 Vidalia onion, chopped

4 large carrots, peeled and chopped

4 celery stalks, chopped

4 garlic cloves, minced

8 ounces cremini mushrooms, thinly sliced

1 cup wild rice

6 cups Classic Vegetable Broth (page 22) or Mushroom Broth (page 29)

1 teaspoon ground sage

¾ teaspoon dried thyme

¾ teaspoon dried rosemary

3 tablespoons butter

¼ cup all-purpose flour

¾ cup whole milk

Salt

Black pepper

1. In a large pot, heat the olive oil over medium-high heat. Add the onion, carrots, and celery and cook until the onion is translucent and the vegetables are tender, 5 to 7 minutes. Add the garlic and cook until fragrant, 1 to 2 minutes.

2. Reduce the heat to medium. Add the mushrooms and cook until they are tender, 5 to 7 minutes. Don't rush this step! The mushrooms will release their moisture and become tender.

3. Add the rice, broth, sage, thyme, and rosemary. Bring to a boil, then reduce to a simmer, and cook for 1½ to 2 hours, until the rice is tender, stirring occasionally.

4. In a small saucepan, melt the butter. Whisk in the flour until fully combined, 1 to 2 minutes. Slowly whisk in the milk until it becomes a smooth and thickened sauce.

5. Mix the creamy mixture into the soup and stir to combine. Season with salt and pepper to taste.

Ingredient tip: Did you know wild rice is not technically a rice, but an aquatic grass? It has a chewy outer sheath that holds the nutrient-dense grain inside, and it grows in shallow water. Many varieties of wild rice have become popular for their high antioxidant, protein, minerals, vitamins, and dietary fiber content.

Continued

Substitution tip: Wild rice does take longer to cook. To trim down on time, look for a whole-grain or wild rice blend.

Per serving: Calories: 290; Fat: 17g; Protein: 6g; Cholesterol: 25mg; Sodium: 440mg; Carbohydrates: 29g; Fiber: 6g

Creamy Pea Soup

SERVES 4 | **PREP TIME** 10 MINUTES | **COOK TIME** 20 MINUTES

Even when made with frozen peas, this soup has fresh-from-the-garden flavor that you can enjoy any season. With just a few flavorful ingredients, this recipe comes together in under 30 minutes. Change it up each time you make it with different toppings to add unique textures and flavors.

GLUTEN-FREE,
DAIRY-FREE, VEGAN,
QUICK PREP, FAST,
FREEZER FRIENDLY

2 tablespoons olive oil

1 medium white onion, diced

2 garlic cloves, crushed

2 cups frozen garden peas

1¾ cups Classic Vegetable
  Broth (see page 22)

¼ cup full-fat coconut milk

Salt

Black pepper

Optional toppings

Thinly sliced radishes

Pomegranate seeds

Balsamic glaze

Mint leaves

Coconut milk (not included
  in nutrition information)

1. Heat the olive oil in a large pot over medium heat. Sauté onion for about 5 minutes, until soft and translucent. Add the garlic and sauté for an additional 1 to 2 minutes, until fragrant.

2. Add frozen peas and vegetable broth.

3. Bring to a boil, then reduce the heat to a simmer and let simmer for 10 minutes.

4. Remove from the heat. Add the coconut milk and, using an immersion blender, blend until smooth.

5. Season with salt and black pepper to taste.

6. Top with preferred optional toppings.

Freezing tip: Freeze the soup without the toppings and add them after the soup is defrosted and heated (see page 18 for thawing and reheating tips).

Ingredient tip: Garden peas are also sometimes called sweet peas or English peas. These peas are sweet and may be eaten raw or cooked and are the commonly sold shelled and frozen.

Per serving: Calories: 160; Fat: 10g; Protein: 4g; Cholesterol: 0mg; Sodium: 170mg; Carbohydrates: 14g; Fiber: 6g

(Dairy-Free) Creamy Tomato Soup

SERVES 6 | PREP TIME 20 MINUTES | **COOK TIME** 30 MINUTES

A creamy tomato soup without an ounce of dairy—how, you ask? The secret ingredient is cashews. Cashews provide the ultimate creaminess when blended into soups. They make this tomato soup so silky and smooth you would never know there isn't dairy in there.

DAIRY-FREE,
FREEZER FRIENDLY,
GLUTEN-FREE, VEGAN

2 tablespoons olive oil

2 onions, chopped

2 celery stalks, chopped

1 tablespoon dried basil

2 garlic cloves, chopped

1 teaspoon salt, plus
    more for seasoning

½ teaspoon black pepper,
    plus more for seasoning

2 (28-ounce) cans no-
    salt-added diced
    tomatoes, with juices

1½ cups water

¾ cup raw cashews

2 tablespoons tomato paste

1. Heat the olive oil in a large pot over medium heat. Add the onions, celery, basil, garlic, salt, and pepper and cook, stirring occasionally, until softened, 5 to 7 minutes.

2. Stir in the tomatoes with their juices, water, cashews, and tomato paste. Bring to a boil, then lower the heat to medium-low and simmer, stirring occasionally, until the soup begins to thicken, 20 to 30 minutes.

3. Allow to cool slightly, for about 15 minutes, then purée in three batches until smooth, transferring the soup to a pot or storage container as it is puréed.

4. Season with additional salt and pepper to taste. Reheat over medium-low heat before serving.

Ingredient tip: Using raw cashews is key. They are naturally smooth and create a creamy consistency when blended into the soup. Cashews contain zinc, which plays a vital role in strengthening the immune system against microbial infections and healing wounds.

Freezer-friendly tip: Have leftover tomato paste? Pre-portion individual tablespoons on a pan lined with wax paper, freeze, then store in a glass container.

Per serving: Calories: 240; Fat: 12g; Protein: 8g; Cholesterol: 0mg; Sodium: 710mg; Carbohydrates: 31g; Fiber: 7g

Creamy Butternut Squash Soup

SERVES 6 | PREP TIME 20 MINUTES | **COOK TIME** 45 MINUTES

We use a few plant-based superstars like cashews and miso to give this thick and delicious soup its flavor and velvety texture.

FREEZER FRIENDLY,
GLUTEN-FREE,
VEGETARIAN

2 tablespoons olive oil

1 large onion, chopped

3 garlic cloves, minced

3 large carrots, peeled
  and diced

1½ tablespoons
  garam masala

⅛ teaspoon nutmeg

2 tablespoons white miso

½ cup raw cashews

1 large butternut squash,
  chopped (about 6 cups)

2 apples, peeled and diced
  (preferably a sweet
  variety like Honeycrisp,
  Gala, Pink Lady)

4 cups Classic Vegetable
  Broth (page 22)

2 cups water

Salt

Black pepper

2 tablespoons plain kefir
  or yogurt (optional)

1. In a large pot, heat the olive oil over medium-high heat. Add the onion, garlic, and carrots. Sauté for 3 to 5 minutes, until the onion starts to become translucent.

2. Add the garam masala and nutmeg. Stir to coat the vegetables.

3. Stir in the miso, cashews, butternut squash, and apples. Stir to combine. Add the broth and water, covering the vegetables. (Use more water, if needed.)

4. Simmer the soup for 30 minutes, until the squash is tender.

5. In batches, transfer the soup to a blender. Blend until smooth. If the soup is too thick, add more water. Season with salt and pepper to taste.

6. Pour the soup into bowls and drizzle with the kefir, if using.

Ingredient tip: Don't want to peel and chop a fresh butternut squash? Use frozen! Frozen is just as nutritionally dense as fresh produce as it is frozen at its peak of ripeness.

Flavor boost: Miso adds a savory flavor to foods that satisfies what is now known as "umami," or our fifth taste sensation.

Per serving: Calories: 250; Fat: 10g; Protein: 5g; Cholesterol: 0mg; Sodium: 240mg; Carbohydrates: 38g; Fiber: 7g

Roasted Red Pepper Bisque

SERVES 4 | PREP TIME 10 MINUTES | **COOK TIME** 20 MINUTES

The use of both roasted red peppers and fresh bell peppers adds layers of flavors. Using light coconut milk gives a creamy element with a hint of sweetness and transforms this soup into a creamy bisque.

DAIRY-FREE,
FREEZER FRIENDLY,
GLUTEN-FREE, QUICK
PREP, VEGAN

1 (12-ounce) jar roasted
   red peppers, drained

1 red bell pepper, diced

1 tablespoon olive oil

2 garlic cloves, minced

2 cups Classic Vegetable
   Broth (page 22)

1 (15-ounce) can light
   coconut milk

½ teaspoon cayenne pepper

¼ teaspoon ground mustard

1 teaspoon red pepper flakes

Salt

Black pepper

Fresh cilantro, for garnish

1. Combine the roasted red peppers, bell pepper, olive oil, and garlic in a large stockpot or Dutch oven. Sauté over medium-high heat until fragrant, then add the broth, coconut milk, cayenne, mustard, and red pepper flakes. Bring to a simmer and cook for 5 minutes.

2. Use an immersion blender, or transfer the soup to a high-speed blender, and blend until smooth. Transfer the blended soup back to the pot and simmer for 10 minutes more, stirring occasionally. Season with salt and pepper to taste.

3. Garnish with cilantro and serve.

Ingredient tip: You can buy roasted red peppers, but if you want to do it yourself, set your oven to broil. Coat fresh bell peppers with olive oil and place them on a parchment paper–lined baking sheet. Broil 10 minutes, rotating every 2 to 3 minutes as the pepper begins to blister. Remove from oven and allow to cool, then slice off the stems and remove the skin (it should peel away easily). Slice or chop and continue on to the recipe.

Per serving: Calories: 200; Fat: 10g; Protein: 4g; Cholesterol: 0mg; Sodium: 250mg; Carbohydrates: 22g; Fiber: 4g

"Cheesy" Broccoli Soup

SERVES 6 | PREP TIME 20 MINUTES | **COOK TIME** 1 HOUR

Chapter 3 includes the classic broccoli cheddar soup (see page 50) recipe. For this variation, we added in a few twists, making it completely plant-based while still packing in a lot of cheesy and delicious flavors. Let's see if you can taste the difference!

DAIRY-FREE,
GLUTEN-FREE, VEGAN

1 pound broccoli florets
  with stems

2 tablespoons olive oil

1 large onion, chopped

1 large carrot, peeled
  and chopped

2 celery stalks, chopped

3 garlic cloves, minced

½ cup nutritional yeast

1 teaspoon smoked paprika

1 Yukon gold potato,
  peeled and chopped

2 cups cauliflower florets

½ cup raw cashews

10 cups Classic Vegetable
  Broth (page 22)

Salt

Black pepper

1. Remove the broccoli florets from the stems. Chop the stems and set aside. Chop the broccoli into small florets and set aside.

2. In a large pot, heat the olive oil over medium-high heat. Sauté the onion, carrot, celery, and broccoli stems, until the onion is translucent and the vegetables are tender, 5 to 7 minutes. Add the garlic and sauté until fragrant, 1 to 2 minutes.

3. Add the nutritional yeast and paprika. Stir to coat the vegetables.

4. Add the potato, cauliflower, cashews, and broth. Stir to combine. Bring to a boil, then reduce to a simmer and cook for 20 to 30 minutes, until the potatoes and cauliflower are fork tender.

5. Working in batches if needed, transfer the soup carefully to a blender and blend until very smooth.

6. Return the mixture to the pot. If the soup is too thick, add water until a desired consistency is reached. Add in the reserved broccoli florets and stir into the soup.

7. Simmer the soup for an additional 10 minutes until broccoli is cooked through.

8. Season with salt and pepper to taste. Top with additional nutritional yeast, if desired.

Continued

"Cheesy" Broccoli Soup *Continued*

Ingredient tip: Nutritional yeast—or nooch as some like to call it—is a lesser-known ingredient that could become your dairy-free secret ingredient. Nutritional yeast is a type of deactivated yeast (unlike typical baker's yeast which foams up and expands). It is a vegan-friendly source of complete protein, B vitamins, and minerals. Use it to replace Parmesan cheese in recipes as it adds a cheesy and nutty flavor profile.

Flavor boost: Smoked paprika, often called pimenton or smoked Spanish paprika, is made from peppers that are smoked and dried over oak fires. This process gives the red powder a rich, smoky flavor.

Per serving: Calories: 260; Fat: 10g; Protein: 11g; Cholesterol: 0mg; Sodium: 330mg; Carbohydrates: 34g; Fiber: 9g

Creamy Roasted Cauliflower Soup

SERVES 4 | **PREP TIME** 10 MINUTES | **COOK TIME** 30 MINUTES

Cauliflower, in our opinion, is the perfect base for a creamy blended soup. It has a mild flavor that serves as a launchpad for other fun flavor pairings. Plus, when roasted, it takes on a subtle sweetness that complements the other flavors of the herbs and crispy chickpeas. Just try to resist snacking on the florets you reserved for toppings!

GLUTEN-FREE, QUICK PREP, VEGETARIAN

1 large cauliflower head, chopped into florets

4 garlic cloves, minced

2 tablespoons olive oil, divided

2 teaspoons ground cumin, divided

2 teaspoons red pepper flakes, divided

1 (15-ounce) can chickpeas, drained and patted dry

1 large onion, diced

3 cups Classic Vegetable Broth (page 22)

14 ounces silken tofu, drained

½ cup whole milk

Salt

Black pepper

Fresh thyme or rosemary, for garnish

1. Preheat the oven to 400°F. Prepare two baking sheets by spraying with nonstick spray or lining with parchment paper.

2. In a mixing bowl, combine the cauliflower florets with the minced garlic, half of the olive oil, cumin, and red pepper flakes. Toss to coat, then spread in a single layer on the first baking sheet. Bake on the upper or middle rack of your oven for 25 minutes, flipping once halfway through if desired for even browning.

3. In the same mixing bowl, toss the chickpeas with the remaining olive oil, cumin, and red pepper flakes. Arrange in a single layer on the second baking sheet. Add to the oven on the middle or lower rack and roast while the cauliflower finishes cooking. Remove both baking sheets at the same time when cook time is complete.

4. Meanwhile, add the onions to a large stockpot or Dutch oven. Add the broth and bring to a simmer.

5. When the cauliflower and chickpeas are finished, remove from oven. Reserve all of the chickpeas and a third of the roasted cauliflower. Add the remaining cauliflower and tofu to the pot and stir to combine. The tofu will start to naturally break apart on its own.

Continued

6. Use an immersion blender to blend to a smooth consistency. Add the milk, then pulse again to combine.

7. Transfer to serving bowls and top with the roasted cauliflower and crispy chickpeas. Season with salt and pepper to taste. Add additional red pepper flakes if desired and garnish with thyme.

Ingredient tip: Silken tofu is a plant-based protein that can help thicken soups and give them a creamy consistency. Tofu is rich in both potassium and calcium: two minerals that are great for bone health and preventing osteoporosis.

Per serving: Calories: 310; Fat: 13g; Protein: 15g; Cholesterol: <5mg; Sodium: 380mg; Carbohydrates: 37g; Fiber: 10g

Spicy Coconut-Pumpkin Soup

SERVES 6 | **PREP TIME** 15 MINUTES | **COOK TIME** 30 MINUTES

This soup will hit all your taste buds with flavor. Temper the amount of spice to your liking, but the coconut milk will help mellow the heat. The fresh lemongrass adds a pop of freshness and some compounds in it are known antioxidants.

DAIRY-FREE,
FREEZER FRIENDLY,
GLUTEN-FREE, VEGAN

1 tablespoon olive oil

1 medium onion, diced

4 garlic cloves, minced

2 tablespoons red
    curry paste

1 teaspoon ground cumin

1 teaspoon ground ginger

1 lemongrass stalk, grated

5 cups Classic Vegetable
    Broth (page 22)

1 (13.5-ounce) can light
    coconut milk

2 (15-ounce) cans
    pumpkin purée

Salt

Black pepper

Chopped cilantro, pumpkin
    seeds (pepitas), and
    additional coconut milk,
    for topping (optional)

1. In a large pot, heat the olive oil over medium-high heat. Add the onion and sauté until tender and translucent, 5 to 7 minutes. Add the garlic, red curry paste, cumin, ginger, and lemongrass, stirring to coat the onions.

2. Add the broth and bring to a boil, then reduce to a simmer. Using an immersion blender, blend the soup until smooth. Alternatively, using a blender, blend the soup in batches until smooth and return to the pot. Reduce the heat to a simmer.

3. Whisk in the coconut milk and pumpkin purée. Simmer for 5 minutes.

4. Season with salt and pepper to taste. Top with cilantro, pumpkin seeds, and a swirl of coconut milk, if using.

Flavor boost: To adjust the heat, add or subtract the amount of red curry paste. You will most likely find red curry paste in the international section in the grocery store.

Ingredient tip: Be sure to use pure pumpkin purée, not pumpkin pie filling. Don't be fooled as the cans look very similar sitting next to each other on grocery store shelves.

Continued

Spicy Coconut-Pumpkin Soup *Continued*

Flavor boost: Lemongrass, a native plant of Southeast Asia and Africa, is used in dishes for its fresh lemon-like aroma. Look for it in the produce aisle, near the fresh herbs. You can also use lemon zest to replicate lemongrass's herbal notes, but the extra zip of tanginess is found in the lemongrass itself.

Per serving: Calories: 150; Fat: 7g; Protein: 3g; Cholesterol: 0mg; Sodium: 240mg; Carbohydrates: 17g; Fiber: 7g

Curry, Carrot, Apple Soup

SERVES 10 | PREP TIME 20 MINUTES | **COOK TIME** 40 MINUTES

This soup is like a big hug—warm, comforting, and so satisfying for the body and soul. This vibrant and velvety soup has flavor complexity from the curry powder. The combination of spices in curry powder also supplies you with potent antioxidants. This mixture of spices can help improve your digestive system and improve your gut health.

DAIRY-FREE,
FREEZER FRIENDLY,
GLUTEN-FREE, VEGAN

1 tablespoon olive oil

1 large onion, chopped

1 leek, halved and sliced

2 celery stalks, chopped

2 tablespoons curry powder

6 large carrots, peeled
  and diced

3 large Honeycrisp apples,
  peeled and chopped

1 bay leaf

6 cups Classic Vegetable
  Broth (page 22)

Salt

Black pepper

1. In a large pot, heat the olive oil over medium-high heat. Add the onion, leek, and celery. Sauté until the onion is translucent and the vegetables are tender, 5 to 7 minutes.

2. Add the curry powder and stir to coat the vegetables.

3. Add the carrots, apples, bay leaf, and broth. Stir well to combine. Bring to a boil, then reduce to a simmer and cover with a lid. Cook for 25 minutes until the carrots and apples are tender.

4. Remove the bay leaf from the soup and discard.

5. Using an immersion blender, blend the soup until smooth and creamy. Alternatively, in small batches blend the soup in a blender and transfer back to the pot.

6. Season with salt and pepper to taste.

Ingredient swap: Use any sweet apple variety like Gala, McIntosh, or Fuji apples.

Flavor boost: Curry powder is a mixture of finely ground spices such as turmeric, ginger, and coriander. That flavor combination adds a warmness to the recipe.

Per serving: Calories: 150; Fat: 3g; Protein: 2g; Cholesterol: 0mg; Sodium: 230mg; Carbohydrates: 30g; Fiber: 7g

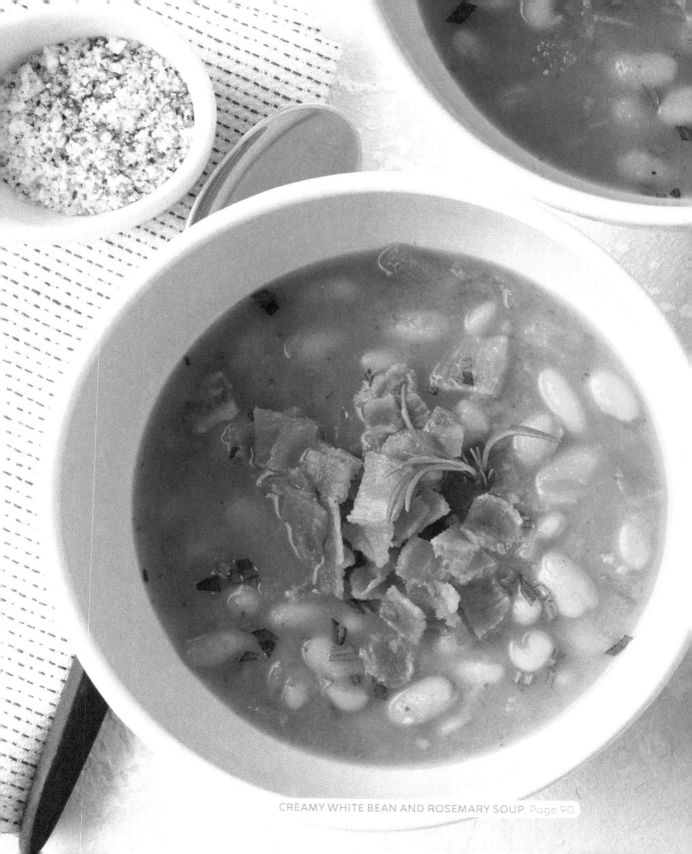

CREAMY WHITE BEAN AND ROSEMARY SOUP, Page 90

5

Grain and Bean Soups

Grains and beans are nutrition powerhouses for so many reasons. They fill us up and fuel us on busy days, providing a good source of gut- and heart-healthy fiber and plant-based protein. One of the challenges with plant-based soups is building deep flavor, so be sure to check the recipe notes for ingredients like nutritional yeast, miso, and Parmesan cheese rinds that serve to create savory umami flavor. Many of these soups are also freezer friendly, so clear some room and store extra portions so you'll always have a good-for-you meal handy when life gets hectic!

Bean and Barley Soup

SERVES 8 | PREP TIME 10 MINUTES | **COOK TIME** 30 MINUTES

You will not miss the meat in this hearty veggie-packed bean and barley soup. This recipe uses quick barley to cut down on cooking time. Quick barley is a type of barley flake that cooks in about 10 minutes, because it has been partially cooked and dried during the flake-rolling process. If you can't find quick barley, sub in regular barley. Simply cook it separately, according to package directions and add it in at the end.

FREEZER FRIENDLY,
VEGETARIAN,
QUICK PREP

2 tablespoons olive oil

2 medium onions, chopped

2 fennel bulbs, cored
  and chopped

8 garlic cloves, minced

1 teaspoon dried basil

½ teaspoon dried oregano

2 (15-ounce) cans no-salt-
  added cannellini beans,
  drained and rinsed

1 (28-ounce) can fire-
  roasted diced tomatoes

12 cups Classic Vegetable
  Broth (page 22)

1½ cups quick-cooking barley

4 cups chopped stemmed
  Swiss chard

Salt

Black pepper

Grated Parmesan cheese,
  for topping (optional)

1. In a large pot, heat the olive oil over medium-high heat. Add the onions and fennel; sauté until the onions are translucent and the vegetables are tender, 5 to 7 minutes. Add the garlic and cook until fragrant, 1 to 2 minutes.

2. Add the basil and oregano. Stir to coat the vegetables.

3. In a small bowl, mash 1 cup of the white beans with the back of a fork, keeping the remaining beans whole.

4. Stir in the mashed beans, whole beans, tomatoes, broth, and barley. Bring to a boil, then reduce to a simmer. Cook for 15 to 20 minutes, until barley is tender.

5. Stir in the Swiss chard and cook until wilted.

6. Season with salt and pepper to taste. Top with Parmesan cheese, if using.

Flavor boost: Raw or cooked, fennel has a faint flavor of licorice or anise, adding a unique depth of flavor to this recipe.

Substitution tip: Any leafy green will work well with this recipe. Try using baby spinach or kale in place of Swiss chard.

Per serving: Calories: 370; Fat: 4.5g; Protein: 15g; Cholesterol: 0mg; Sodium: 490mg; Carbohydrates: 72g; Fiber: 17g

Vegetable Lentil Soup

SERVES 8 | **PREP TIME** 15 MINUTES | **COOK TIME** 45 MINUTES

This vegan-friendly soup can help you meet your daily amount of veggies for the day! Lentils are plant protein superstars and are also high in fiber and complex carbohydrates for long-lasting energy.

DAIRY-FREE, FREEZER FRIENDLY, GLUTEN-FREE, VEGAN

2 tablespoons olive oil

1 medium onion, diced

2 large carrots, peeled and chopped

5 garlic cloves, minced

2 teaspoons ground cumin

1 teaspoon smoked paprika

½ teaspoon dried thyme

¼ teaspoon red pepper flakes

1 cup green lentils

1 (15-ounce) can chickpeas, rinsed and drained

2 (15-ounce) cans fire-roasted tomatoes

4 cups Classic Vegetable Broth (page 22)

3 cups chopped baby spinach

Salt

Black pepper

1. In a large pot, heat the olive oil over medium–high heat. Add the onion and carrots. Sauté until the onions are translucent and the vegetables are tender, 5 to 7 minutes. Add the garlic and cook until fragrant, 1 to 2 minutes.

2. Add the cumin, paprika, thyme, and red pepper flakes. Stir the herbs and spices to coat the vegetables.

3. Add the lentils, chickpeas, tomatoes, and broth. Bring to a boil, then reduce to a simmer. Simmer for 30 to 35 minutes, until the lentils are tender.

4. Transfer 3 cups of the soup to a blender and purée until smooth. (Get an even mixture of veggies and broth.) Add the puréed soup back into the pot.

5. Add the spinach and stir until it has wilted.

6. Season with salt and pepper to taste.

Substitution tip: Switch up your greens! Both kale and Swiss chard work with this recipe, too.

Flavor boost: Smoked paprika uses chilies that are smoke-dried and then crushed. Smoked paprika adds a smokiness to this recipe.

Per serving: Calories: 210; Fat: 5g; Protein: 10g; Cholesterol: 0mg; Sodium: 490mg; Carbohydrates: 33g; Fiber: 12g

Lemon Sorghum Vegetable Soup

SERVES 8 | PREP TIME 10 MINUTES | **COOK TIME** 25 MINUTES

Adding the lemon rind to the simmering broth infuses the lemon flavor in each bite. Sorghum is an extremely versatile grain that you can use like rice or quinoa. Sorghum contains 10 percent protein and nearly 75 percent complex carbohydrates, and it is rich in B-complex vitamins to help you feel fuller longer and power you through your day. However, if you can't find sorghum, any whole grain (such as quinoa, freekeh, or barley) will work in this recipe. Cook time may vary depending on the grain.

FAST, GLUTEN-FREE, QUICK PREP, VEGETARIAN

2 tablespoons olive oil

1 large onion, diced

2 large carrots, peeled and diced

2 celery stalks, diced

4 garlic cloves, minced

2 teaspoons herbs de Provence

¼ teaspoon red pepper flakes

1 cup sorghum

2 lemons, zested and juiced

1 (15-ounce) can petite diced tomatoes, drained

8 cups Classic Vegetable Broth (page 22)

3 cups chopped baby kale

Salt

Black pepper

Chopped chives and crumbled feta cheese, for topping (optional)

1. In a large pot, heat the olive oil over medium-high heat. Add the onion, carrots, and celery, and sauté until the onion is translucent and the vegetables are tender, 5 to 7 minutes. Add the garlic and cook until fragrant, 1 to 2 minutes.

2. Add the herbs de Provence, red pepper flakes, sorghum, lemon zest, and lemon juice. Stir to combine. Add the lemon rind to the pot to infuse even more lemon flavor.

3. Add the tomatoes and broth. Bring to a boil, then reduce to a simmer. Simmer for 15 minutes.

4. Stir in the kale and cook until wilted. Season with salt and pepper to taste.

5. Top with chives and feta cheese, if using.

Substitution tip: Don't have herbs de Provence seasoning mix? You can use an Italian seasoning mix or dried thyme instead.

Per serving: Calories: 170; Fat: 4.5g; Protein: 5g; Cholesterol: 0mg; Sodium: 280mg; Carbohydrates: 31g; Fiber: 5g

Taco Soup

SERVES 8 | PREP TIME 20 MINUTES | **COOK TIME** 40 MINUTES

Soups on for Taco Tuesday! Keep it mild or make it spicy, depending on what your taste buds prefer. Eating vegetables every day is important for optimal health. They provide essential vitamins, minerals, and other nutrients, such as antioxidants and fiber. Research consistently shows that people who eat the most vegetables have the lowest risk of many diseases, including cancer and heart disease.

GLUTEN-FREE,
VEGETARIAN

1 tablespoon olive oil

1 large onion, chopped

2 red bell peppers, chopped

3 carrots, peeled
  and chopped

3 garlic cloves, chopped

3 zucchini, chopped

1 cup frozen corn

2 tablespoons ground cumin

2 teaspoons chili powder

1 (28-ounce) can fire-roasted
  crushed tomatoes

5 cups Classic Vegetable
  Broth (page 22)

1 (14.5-ounce) can black
  beans, rinsed and drained

1 (7-ounce) can green chiles

Salt

Black pepper

½ cup shredded
  cheddar cheese

Lime wedges, chopped
  cilantro, cubed avocado,
  for topping (optional)

1. In a large pot, heat the olive oil over medium-high heat. Add the onion, bell peppers, and carrots. Sauté until the onion is translucent and the vegetables are tender, 5 to 7 minutes. Add the garlic and cook until fragrant, 1 to 2 minutes.

2. Add the zucchini and corn. Add the cumin and chili powder. Stir to coat the vegetables with spices.

3. Add the tomatoes and broth. Stir to combine. Bring to a boil, then reduce to a simmer. Cook for 30 minutes, until the vegetables are tender.

4. Stir in the black beans and green chiles.

5. Season with salt and pepper to taste. Top with cheddar cheese and other toppings, if using.

Ingredient tip: For less spice, remove the green chiles.

Flavor boost: Using fire-roasted tomatoes adds depth of flavor in this soup by providing a hint of smokiness.

Substitution tip: You can add 1 pound of beef or turkey to this soup for the meat lovers. Sauté the meat in a pan separately and add it into the soup. If adding meat, you will need to increase the liquid by using additional broth or water.

Per serving: Calories: 190; Fat: 5g; Protein: 8g; Cholesterol: 5mg; Sodium: 640mg; Carbohydrates: 30g; Fiber: 9g

Classic Three-Bean Chili

SERVES 8 | **PREP TIME** 10 MINUTES | **COOK TIME** 50 MINUTES

There are many traditional versions of chili, ranging from the classic chili con carne to plant-based versions. Traditionalists often exclude beans and grains to focus on the blend of meats, spices, and red or green chiles. Due to its hearty nature, chili is rarely seen as a healthful food, but we prefer to think of it as something better than the sum of its parts. It provides valuable nutrition (protein, carbs, fat, and fiber) and can be a budget-friendly option, too. If you're conscious of the impact of your food choices, beans and legumes are also among the most environmentally-friendly food choices out there, so don't be shy about adding more of them to your chili!

GLUTEN-FREE, QUICK
PREP, VEGETARIAN

1 tablespoon olive oil

1 large onion, chopped

1 large red bell pepper, chopped

1 large yellow bell pepper, chopped

1 jalapeño, seeded and finely chopped

1 tablespoon garlic powder

2 teaspoons ground cumin

1 teaspoon chili powder

1 (15-ounce) can red kidney beans, drained and rinsed

1 (15-ounce) can black beans, drained and rinsed

1 (15-ounce) can pinto beans, drained and rinsed

1 cup frozen corn, thawed

2 (15-ounce) cans petite diced tomatoes, with juices

1. In a large pot, heat the olive oil over medium-high heat. Add the onion, bell peppers, and jalapeño, and sauté until the onion is translucent and vegetables are tender, 5 to 7 minutes.

2. Add the garlic powder, cumin, and chili powder. Stir to coat vegetables with spices.

3. Add the kidney beans, black beans, pinto beans, corn, tomatoes, and broth. Heat to a low simmer and simmer for 40 minutes.

4. Adjust the consistency by simmering the chili for longer to thicken or add more broth to thin.

1 cup Classic Vegetable
   Broth (page 22)

Salt

Black pepper

Sliced avocado, scallions,
   Greek yogurt, shredded
   cheddar cheese, for
   topping (optional)

5. Season with salt and pepper to taste. Top with avocado, scallions, Greek yogurt, and cheddar cheese,
   if using.

Flavor boost: For a spicy/smoky flavor, add a small can of
chipotle chiles in adobo sauce. Look for it in the international
aisle or near the taco ingredients in the grocery store.

Ingredient tip: Wear gloves when seeding and chopping the
jalapeño to avoid contact with capsaicin, which can cause
irritation.

Per serving: Calories: 230; Fat: 3g; Protein: 12g;
Cholesterol: 0mg; Sodium: 560mg; Carbohydrates: 41g;
Fiber: 12g

Pasta e Fagioli

SERVES 6 | **PREP TIME** 15 MINUTES | **COOK TIME** 20 MINUTES

The word pasta fazool *(or pasta e fagioli) originated in Italy and means "pasta and beans." It was once considered a peasant dish because it's made of inexpensive ingredients, but now it has many variations. Often people add bacon or pancetta, but we're fans of this plant-based version that truly plays up the beans and pasta. Be sure to finely dice the vegetables so they don't outshine the main ingredients.*

VEGETARIAN

1 tablespoon olive oil

1 medium onion, finely diced

1 large carrot, peeled and finely diced

2 celery stalks, finely diced

5 garlic cloves, minced

½ tablespoon dried rosemary

1 teaspoon dried thyme

1 teaspoon dried oregano

¼ teaspoon red pepper flakes

1 bay leaf

4 cups Classic Vegetable Broth (page 22) or Chicken Broth (page 24)

1 (15-ounce) can crushed tomatoes

1 cup water

1 cup whole-wheat ditalini pasta

2 (15-ounce) cans cannellini beans, drained and rinsed

Salt

Black pepper

Grated Parmesan cheese (optional)

1. In a large pot, heat the olive oil over medium-high heat. Add the onion, carrots, and celery, and sauté until the onion is translucent and the vegetables are tender, 4 to 6 minutes. Add the garlic and cook until fragrant, 1 to 2 minutes.

2. Add the rosemary, thyme, oregano, red pepper flakes, and bay leaf. Stir the herbs and spices with the vegetables to coat.

3. Add the broth, tomatoes, and water. Bring to a rapid boil.

4. Stir in the pasta and beans. Reduce the heat to medium for a low boil. Cook for 6 to 8 minutes, or until the pasta is al dente, stirring occasionally.

5. Remove the bay leaf. Season with salt and pepper to taste. Top with Parmesan cheese, if using.

Substitution tip: Any small-shaped pasta will work. Adjust the cook time, if necessary, so the pasta cooks until al dente.

Flavor boost: Looking for a little more heat? Add an extra pinch of red pepper flakes.

Per serving: Calories: 300; Fat: 3.5g; Protein: 14g; Cholesterol: 0mg; Sodium: 280mg; Carbohydrates: 56g; Fiber: 11g

Tuscan Bean Soup

SERVES 8 | PREP TIME 15 MINUTES | **COOK TIME** 35 MINUTES

This hearty and healthy rustic soup is sure to impress and incredibly easy to make. Pearled couscous are small balls of toasted semolina flour. If you can't find it, simply swap out a different grain to your liking. Cooking time may vary depending on the time needed to cook the substituted grain.

VEGETARIAN

2 tablespoons olive oil

1 large onion, finely chopped

3 medium carrots, peeled and finely chopped

3 celery stalks, finely chopped

4 garlic cloves, minced

2 teaspoons dried oregano

1 teaspoon dried basil

1 tablespoon tomato paste

1 (15-ounce) can petite diced tomatoes, with juices

8 cups Classic Vegetable Broth (page 22)

1 (3-inch) Parmesan rind

1 cup pearled couscous

1 (15-ounce) can cannellini beans, drained and rinsed

3 cups shredded stemmed lacinato kale

Salt

Black pepper

½ cup pesto

1. In large pot, heat the olive oil over medium-high heat. Add the onion, carrots, and celery. Sauté until the onion is translucent and the vegetables are tender, 5 to 7 minutes. Add the garlic and cook until fragrant, 1 to 2 minutes.

2. Add the oregano, basil, and tomato paste. Stir to coat the vegetables.

3. Add the tomatoes, broth, Parmesan rind, and couscous. Bring to a boil, then reduce to a simmer and cook for 15 to 20 minutes, until the couscous is tender.

4. Remove the Parmesan rind, if it hasn't disintegrated. Add the beans and kale. Cook until the kale has wilted. Season with salt and pepper to taste.

5. Pour the soup into bowls and top with the pesto.

Substitution tip: Lacinato or dino kale is a fun ingredient to cook with, but if you can't find it, look for other varieties of kale, or swap it out for Swiss or rainbow chard.

Flavor boost: Why add a Parmesan cheese rind into soup? The rind will soften, and the flavors of the cheese will infuse throughout the soup.

Per serving: Calories: 250; Fat: 4.5g; Protein: 10g; Cholesterol: <5mg; Sodium: 380mg; Carbohydrates: 42g; Fiber: 7g

"Creamy" Italian Quinoa Soup

SERVES 6 | **PREP TIME** 10 MINUTES | **COOK TIME** 40 MINUTES

This soup is simple to make using a cashew "cream" instead of a dairy-based cream. Nutritional yeast plus miso paste creates a rich flavor that pairs well with this tomato-based soup. If you're cooking this during the colder months, dried herbs are an affordable and reliable option, but if you're cooking in the summertime, feel free to swap in fresh herbs and adjust the seasoning to your tastes (generally you can use a 3:1 ratio of fresh to dried herbs). To make a dairy version, replace the "cream" with ½ cup of half-and-half.

DAIRY-FREE,
GLUTEN-FREE, QUICK
PREP, VEGAN

For the soup

2 tablespoons olive oil

1 large yellow onion, diced

2 large carrots, chopped

2 celery stalks, sliced

3 garlic cloves, minced

Salt

Black pepper

1 (15-ounce) can chickpeas, drained and rinsed

⅓ cup white or tricolor quinoa

1 (14.5-ounce) can crushed tomatoes

1 (6-ounce) can tomato paste

4 cups Classic Vegetable Broth (page 22)

1 tablespoon dried Italian herbs

4 cups fresh spinach

To make the soup

1. Heat the olive oil in a large stockpot or Dutch oven over medium-high heat. Add the onion, carrots, and celery and sauté for about 5 minutes, until the onion becomes translucent. Add the garlic and cook 1 minute more. Season with salt and pepper to taste.

2. Add the chickpeas and quinoa, then cover with the tomatoes, tomato paste, and broth. Add the Italian herbs and bring to a boil. Reduce the heat, then simmer, partially covered, for 20 to 25 minutes.

3. Just before serving, fold in the spinach and allow to wilt slightly. Remove from the heat, then stir in the "cream."

To make the "cream"

1. While the soup is cooking, prepare the "cream" by combining the cashews, nutritional yeast, miso paste, and broth in a high-speed blender. Blend on high speed until smooth and creamy.

For the "cream"

½ cup raw, unsalted cashews

2 tablespoons
   nutritional yeast

1 teaspoon miso paste

½ cup warm Classic
   Vegetable Broth (page 22)

Ingredient tip: Miso paste adds a lot of savory flavor to this soup. Look for prepared miso in tubes or tubs in the Asian section or near refrigerated tofu at your grocery store. If you aren't able to find it, it can also be purchased online.

Ingredient tip: Rinsing removes quinoa's natural coating (saponin), which can make it taste bitter or soapy. Although boxed quinoa is often prerinsed, it doesn't hurt to give the seeds an additional rinse at home.

Per serving: Calories: 260; Fat: 9g; Protein: 9g; Cholesterol: 5mg; Sodium: 400mg; Carbohydrates: 38g; Fiber: 9g

Per serving (dairy-free version): Calories: 310; Fat: 12g; Protein: 12g; Cholesterol: 0mg; Sodium: 470mg; Carbohydrates: 42g; Fiber: 10g

Creamy White Bean and Rosemary Soup

SERVES 6 | PREP TIME 10 MINUTES | **COOK TIME** 45 MINUTES

White beans lend a wonderful creamy texture to soups when blended. Since the texture is intended to be chunky, canned beans are fine to use, saving time and energy compared to cooking with dried beans. This thick soup is great paired with crusty bread for dipping or a side salad or sandwich (not reflected in nutrition calculations).

DAIRY-FREE,
FREEZER FRIENDLY,
GLUTEN-FREE,
QUICK PREP

¼ cup olive oil

1 large yellow onion, diced

3 garlic cloves, minced

3 (15-ounce) cans white cannellini or Great Northern beans, drained and rinsed

6 cups Chicken Stock (page 25)

2 large rosemary sprigs, plus more for garnish

Salt

Black pepper

¼ teaspoon cayenne pepper

4 cooked bacon slices, crumbled

1. In a large stockpot, heat the olive oil over medium-high heat. Add the onion and cook for 10 to 15 minutes until its edges begin to caramelize. Add the garlic and cook 1 minute more.

2. Add the beans, stock, rosemary, salt, and pepper. Bring to a boil, then reduce the heat and simmer for 15 to 20 minutes.

3. Carefully transfer half of the contents to a high-speed blender or a small saucepan. Blend to a smooth purée using either a high-speed blender or an immersion blender. Add the cayenne to the purée, then season with salt and pepper to taste.

4. Return the purée to the stockpot and fold to combine.

5. To serve, garnish with fresh rosemary and the crumbled bacon. Serve immediately.

Storage tip: This is freezer friendly if you want to make larger batches for prepped meals to enjoy later. Freeze without the toppings and add later when reheated.

Per serving: Calories: 450; Fat: 15g; Protein: 24g; Cholesterol: 15mg; Sodium: 500mg; Carbohydrates: 57g; Fiber: 11g

Chickpea Noodle Soup

SERVES 6 | PREP TIME 10 MINUTES | **COOK TIME** 20 MINUTES

Chickpeas are a natural replacement for chicken—and not just because of their name! They have a neutral flavor but are protein- and fiber-rich, and they add a creamy texture when cooked with the other ingredients. Fiber is essential for regulating blood sugar as well as for a healthy heart and gut. Nutritional yeast adds savory umami-like flavor, so you won't be missing the flavor that is normally provided by chicken.

DAIRY-FREE, FAST,
QUICK PREP, VEGAN

2 tablespoons olive oil

1 large yellow onion,
   chopped

3 large carrots, sliced

2 celery stalks, sliced

Salt

Black pepper

3 tablespoons
   nutritional yeast

2 teaspoons fresh thyme
   leaves or ¾ teaspoon
   dried thyme

2 garlic cloves, minced

2 bay leaves

6 cups Classic Vegetable
   Broth (page 22)

2 (15-ounce) cans chickpeas,
   drained and rinsed

1 cup ditalini pasta

2 tablespoons fresh parsley

1. Heat the olive oil in a large stockpot or Dutch oven over medium-high heat. Add the onion, carrots, and celery. Season with salt and pepper. Cook, stirring occasionally, until the veggies begin to soften, 5 to 7 minutes.

2. Add the nutritional yeast, thyme, garlic, and bay leaves and cook until fragrant, about 1 minute.

3. Stir in the broth and chickpeas and bring to a boil. Add the pasta and simmer until just tender, 10 to 11 minutes. If desired, leave pasta slightly under-cooked as it will continue cooking once removed from the heat.

4. Remove the bay leaves and stir in the parsley. Season with salt and pepper to taste, then serve immediately.

Substitution tip: Ditalini pasta is a small tube-shaped pasta that is similar in size to the chickpeas and other ingredients in this soup. That makes it easy for serving and slurping, but if needed, you may also use other pastas. Adjust cook time according to package instructions.

Per serving: Calories: 310; Fat: 7g; Protein: 12g; Cholesterol: 0mg; Sodium: 410mg; Carbohydrates: 51g; Fiber: 10g

Golden Lentil Soup

SERVES 6 | PREP TIME 15 MINUTES, 2 HOURS TO SOAK | **COOK TIME** 45 MINUTES

Made with warming spices and protein-packed lentils, this is a meal in a bowl, but we encourage crusty bread for extra dipping. Just ½ cup of cooked lentils provides 15 percent of your daily iron needs! For vegetarians, getting enough iron is particularly challenging. Regularly including lentils in your diet can help boost your iron intake.

DAIRY-FREE,
FREEZER FRIENDLY,
GLUTEN-FREE, VEGAN

½ cup raw cashews

2 cups water

1 ½ tablespoons olive oil

1 large Vidalia onion, diced

3 medium carrots,
  peeled and diced

1 fennel bulb, cored
  and chopped

5 garlic cloves, minced

2 teaspoons ground cumin

2 teaspoons ground turmeric

1 teaspoon dried thyme

¾ cup green lentils, rinsed

1 (14-ounce) can no-salt-
  added diced tomatoes

6 cups Classic Vegetable
  Broth (page 22)

3 cups baby spinach

1 teaspoon balsamic vinegar

Salt

Black pepper

1. Put the cashews in a small bowl and cover with 1½ cups of the water. Let soak for 1 to 2 hours. (For a faster method, cover with boiling water for 30 minutes). Drain and rinse. Add the cashews to a blender with the remaining ½ cup of water. Blend until smooth and creamy. Set aside the cashew cream.

2. In a large pot, heat the olive oil over medium-high heat. Add the onion, carrots, and fennel, and sauté until the onion is translucent and the vegetables are tender, 5 to 7 minutes. Add the garlic and cook until fragrant, 1 to 2 minutes.

3. Add the cumin, turmeric, and thyme. Stir to coat the vegetables.

4. Add the lentils, tomatoes, and broth, stirring to combine. Bring to a boil, reduce to a simmer, and cook for 30 to 35 minutes until the lentils are tender.

5. Stir in the cashew cream, spinach, and vinegar, and cook until the spinach has wilted. Season with salt and pepper to taste.

Storage tip: Leftover soup may thicken after sitting in the refrigerator. Simply thin it out with a little extra broth or water when you reheat it.

Ingredient tip: Be sure to rinse and sort lentils to remove any debris or hidden stones tucked away among the legumes.

Substitution tip: Don't love the strong fennel flavor? Use 3 celery stalks instead.

Per serving: Calories: 250; Fat: 9g; Protein: 11g; Cholesterol: 0mg; Sodium: 370mg; Carbohydrates: 34g; Fiber: 12g

Cuban-Style Black Bean Soup

SERVES 6 | PREP TIME 10 MINUTES | **COOK TIME** 3 HOURS

This beautiful soup features some bold flavors, but the spices in Cuban cuisine are not as pronounced as some other Latin-inspired dishes. For convenience we relied on dried oregano, but if you have fresh available, you can impart a subtly different flavor. Omit the bacon if you prefer a vegetarian soup.

DAIRY-FREE, GLUTEN-FREE, QUICK PREP

½ pound dried black beans

1 bay leaf

6½ cups Classic Vegetable Broth (page 22)

1 tablespoon olive oil

1 large green bell pepper, chopped

1 small yellow onion, chopped

½ tablespoon ground cumin

1 tablespoon dried oregano

2 garlic cloves, minced

½ tablespoon packed brown sugar

Salt

Black pepper

1 ripe avocado, diced

2 scallions, thinly sliced, for topping

½ cup cooked bacon, crumbled (optional)

½ cup chopped fresh cilantro

1. Pick through the dried beans to remove any debris. Place in a large stockpot or Dutch oven with the bay leaf and broth. Bring to a boil.

2. Reduce the heat and simmer for 2½ hours, until the beans are tender, stirring occasionally.

3. Heat the olive oil in a large skillet over medium heat. Add the bell pepper and onion and cook 5 to 6 minutes, or until the onion is translucent.

4. Stir in the cumin, oregano, and garlic and cook 2 minutes more. Remove from the heat, then transfer the veggie mixture to a blender. Add ½ cup of the cooking liquid from the black beans and purée until smooth. Once blended, add the sugar and stir to combine.

5. Add the vegetable mixture to the black beans and simmer for 10 minutes, stirring occasionally. Remove the bay leaf. Season with salt and pepper to taste.

6. Ladle the black beans into serving bowls, then top each bowl with the avocado, scallions, bacon, if using, cilantro, pepitas, and jalapeño. Drizzle with the lime juice and serve immediately.

¼ cup pepitas

1 small jalapeño, seeded
   and minced

1 tablespoon fresh lime juice

Slow cooker option: If you like the convenience of using a slow cooker to cook dried beans instead, you have the option to cook on high for 3 to 4 hours or low for 5 to 6 hours. Follow instructions for the remaining ingredients. Soaking the beans overnight will also speed the cooking process and reduce total stovetop time to about an hour.

Per serving: Calories: 300; Fat: 12g; Protein: 14g; Cholesterol: 5mg; Sodium: 300mg; Carbohydrates: 36g; Fiber: 10g

Kimchi Veggie Soup

SERVES 6 | PREP TIME 10 MINUTES | **COOK TIME** 25 MINUTES

Though this soup is inspired by Asian flavors, it uses familiar vegetables. It's a hearty fall and winter soup, but if Brussels sprouts aren't available, sub in another favorite vegetable. Keep in mind that high heat can damage the beneficial probiotics in kimchi, so allow the soup to cool slightly before adding the kimchi just before serving. Fermented foods such as kimchi can support a healthy gut microbiome.

FAST, QUICK PREP,
VEGETARIAN,
DAIRY-FREE

1 tablespoon sesame oil

½ pound Brussels sprouts, trimmed and shredded

1 medium yellow onion, thinly sliced

2 garlic cloves, grated

1½ tablespoons grated fresh ginger

6 cups Classic Vegetable Broth (page 22)

8 ounces thin rice noodles

1 cup thinly sliced radishes

1 small bunch green or purple kale, stemmed and chopped

4 large eggs

1 cup chopped kimchi, with juices

1 tablespoon low-sodium soy sauce

2 scallions, thinly sliced

Salt

Black pepper

1. Heat the sesame oil in a large stockpot or Dutch oven over medium-high heat. Add the Brussels sprouts and onion and cook until browned and caramelized, about 10 minutes, stirring occasionally.

2. Add the garlic and ginger and stir to combine. Cover with the broth and bring to a low simmer. Add the rice noodles and cook according to package directions. When the noodles have nearly finished cooking, stir in the radishes and kale and allow to wilt. Remove from the heat and allow to cool slightly.

3. Meanwhile, poach the eggs and divide the soup into serving bowls. Top each bowl with one egg, then stir in the kimchi and soy sauce.

4. Garnish with the scallions; serve immediately. Season with salt and pepper to taste.

Ingredient tip: If poaching eggs is too much effort, you can also quick-fry them in a nonstick skillet and add to the top of your bowl. For a prep-ahead option, you can also use hard-boiled eggs. Slice into thin rounds and place on top of your hot soup to allow it to heat through before serving.

Per serving: Calories: 290; Fat: 6g; Protein: 11g; Cholesterol: 125mg; Sodium: 720mg; Carbohydrates: 46g; Fiber: 6g

Vegetarian Moroccan-Style Stew

SERVES 8 | PREP TIME 20 MINUTES | **COOK TIME** 50 MINUTES

This fragrant, spicy stew has a hint of sweetness. It can be served over couscous or accompanied by warm pita bread. Try topping it with a dollop of yogurt. Sweet potatoes are high in both vitamin C and beta-carotene and offer an immunity boost from its powerful combination of nutrients.

GLUTEN-FREE,
VEGETARIAN

2 tablespoons olive oil

1 large onion, chopped

3 medium carrots,
    peeled and chopped

4 garlic cloves, minced

1 large cauliflower head, cut
    into florets (about 4 cups)

1 large sweet potato,
    peeled and cubed

½ tablespoon smoked paprika

½ teaspoon chili powder

1 teaspoon ground coriander

1 teaspoon ground cinnamon

½ teaspoon ground turmeric

1 (28-ounce) can whole
    peeled tomatoes

½ cup chopped dried apricots

4 cups Classic Vegetable
    Broth (page 22)

1 (15-ounce) can chickpeas,
    rinsed and drained

Juice of 1 lemon

Salt

Black pepper

Chopped fresh parsley
    (optional)

¼ cup plain yogurt

1. In a large wide pot, heat the olive oil over medium-high heat. Add the onion and carrots and sauté until the onion is translucent and the vegetables are tender, 5 to 7 minutes. Add the garlic and cook until fragrant, 1 to 2 minutes. Add the cauliflower and sweet potatoes. Stir to combine.

2. Add the paprika, chili powder, coriander, cinnamon, and turmeric. Stir to coat the vegetables. Cook for 5 minutes, stirring occasionally.

3. Add the tomatoes, apricots, and broth. Bring to a boil and cook for 10 minutes. Reduce to a simmer and cook for 25 minutes, or until the vegetables are tender, stirring occasionally.

4. Stir in the chickpeas and lemon juice. Season with salt and pepper to taste.

5. Garnish with parsley and yogurt and serve.

Flavor boost: Moroccan meals typically do not end with dessert. Instead, opt to add pops of sweetness into these savory dishes with dried fruits, like dried apricots.

Per serving: Calories: 200; Fat: 5g; Protein: 7g; Cholesterol: 0mg; Sodium: 420mg; Carbohydrates: 36g; Fiber: 9g

North African-Style Red Lentil Soup

SERVES 6 | PREP TIME 10 MINUTES | **COOK TIME** 30 MINUTES

Red lentils are a blank slate for rich spices and flavors inspired by North Africa. They break down into a thick, creamy consistency all on their own. Don't be shy about stocking up on spices; we think you'll enjoy this soup enough to cook it again and again! This delicious soup offers an extra boost of gut-healthy fiber.

DAIRY-FREE,
FREEZER FRIENDLY,
GLUTEN-FREE,
QUICK PREP , VEGAN

3 tablespoons olive
   oil, divided

1 large yellow onion,
   chopped

Salt

Black pepper

¾ teaspoon ground
   coriander

½ teaspoon ground cumin

¼ teaspoon ground ginger

¼ teaspoon ground
   cinnamon

⅛ teaspoon cayenne pepper

2 tablespoons tomato paste

2 garlic cloves, minced

6 cups Classic Vegetable
   Broth (page 22)

1½ cups red lentils

2 tablespoons lemon juice

1½ teaspoons dried mint

1. Heat 1 tablespoon of the olive oil in a large heavy-bottomed skillet or Dutch oven over medium heat. Add the onion and season with salt and pepper. Cook until the onion is translucent, about 5 minutes.

2. Stir in the coriander, cumin, ginger, cinnamon, and cayenne and cook until fragrant, about 1 minute more. Stir in the tomato paste and garlic, stirring to combine.

3. Add the broth and lentils and bring to a low boil. Cook, uncovered, stirring occasionally, until the lentils are soft and begin to break apart, about 15 minutes.

4. Vigorously whisk the mixture into a coarse blend. If needed, add small amounts of hot water to reach your desired consistency. Stir in the lemon juice, then cover to keep warm.

5. Heat the remaining 2 tablespoons of olive oil in a small saucepan, then remove from the heat and add the mint and paprika.

6. Ladle the soup into bowls. Then drizzle with the spiced oil mixture. Top with the peanuts and cilantro. Serve immediately.

1 teaspoon smoked paprika

½ cup chopped peanuts

Fresh cilantro, for serving

Flavor boost: The flavors of multiple spices need an opportunity to blend together, and the heat of the oil and onion mixture does just that. Take care to not burn the spices though, otherwise the final flavor may carry some off notes. When in doubt, reduce the heat until the broth is added.

Per serving: Calories: 360; Fat: 14g; Protein: 17g; Cholesterol: 0mg; Sodium: 170mg; Carbohydrates: 43g; Fiber: 17g

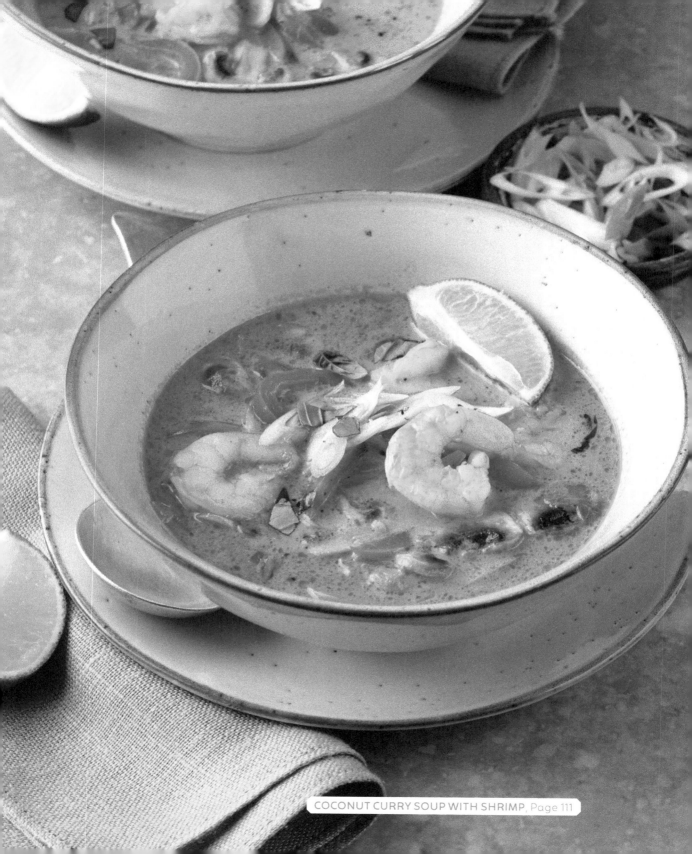

COCONUT CURRY SOUP WITH SHRIMP, Page 111

6

Fish and Shellfish Soups

No matter where you live, there are more seafood options available than ever before. Frozen and canned options are just as nutritious as fresh fish and seafood, and are often more affordable with the same level of quality. Fish and seafood are one of the best sources for omega-3 fatty acids, and most Americans don't consume the recommended two servings a week. These delicious soups and stews highlight some of our favorite ways to use fish and seafood. You'll see global influences, but don't worry, we made sure to keep specialty ingredients to a minimum. You should be able to find these ingredients at most major retailers.

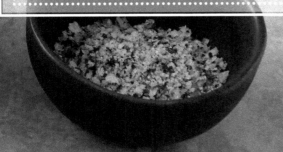

Manhattan Clam Chowder

SERVES 8 | PREP TIME 15 MINUTES | **COOK TIME** 40 MINUTES

Not all clam chowders are created equally. When we think of clam chowder, many think of the New England style creamy version. Looking for something a little lighter? This version uses a brothy tomato base. Lycopene is a powerful antioxidant with many health benefits, including sun protection, improved heart health, and the ability to lower risk of certain types of cancer. More than 80 percent of the lycopene in American diets comes from the consumption of tomato products.

DAIRY-FREE,
GLUTEN-FREE

2 tablespoons olive oil

1 large onion, diced

3 celery stalks, diced

2 green bell peppers, diced

6 garlic cloves, minced

¼ teaspoon red pepper flakes

2 teaspoons dried parsley

2 teaspoons dried thyme

2 bay leaves

2 tablespoons tomato paste

1 large Red Bliss or
   waxy potato, cut
   into small cubes

2 cups clam juice

3 cups Classic Vegetable
   Broth (page 22)

1 (28-ounce) can
   crushed tomatoes

4 (6.5-ounce) cans
   clams, drained, rinsed,
   and minced

Salt

Black pepper

¼ cup chopped fresh parsley

1. In a large pot, heat the olive oil over medium-high heat. Add the onion, celery, and bell peppers and sauté until the onion is translucent and the vegetables are tender, 5 to 7 minutes. Add the garlic and sauté until fragrant, 1 to 2 minutes. Add the red pepper flakes, dried parsley, thyme, bay leaves, and tomato paste and stir to coat the vegetables.

2. Add the potato, clam juice, and broth. Bring to a boil, then reduce to a simmer and cook until the potato is tender, about 10 minutes.

3. Stir in the tomatoes and clams. Simmer for another 5 to 10 minutes.

4. Season with salt and pepper to taste. Garnish with the parsley.

Ingredient tip: Make sure to drain and rinse canned clams, as they tend to have higher amounts of sodium.

Per serving: Calories: 270; Fat: 5g; Protein: 26g; Cholesterol: 45mg; Sodium: 650mg; Carbohydrates: 29g; Fiber: 5g

New England Bay Scallop Chowder

SERVES 6 | PREP TIME 15 MINUTES | **COOK TIME** 35 MINUTES

Here's another variation of a chowder recipe that features bay scallops. This type of bivalve is much smaller than its sea scallop counterpart, usually only about ½-inch wide. They cook quickly, so when searing for flavor, be sure not to overcook them. If you're worried that may happen, skip that step and add toward the end of cooking for a moist cooking method that won't leave them tough or chewy.

GLUTEN-FREE

2 tablespoons olive oil

12 ounces frozen bay scallops, thawed

1 large yellow onion, chopped

2 large white potatoes, peeled and diced

2 celery stalks, chopped

2 (3-ounce) tins smoked oysters

2 bay leaves

4 cups Classic Vegetable Broth (page 22) or seafood stock

2½ cups whole milk

⅛ teaspoon white pepper

¼ teaspoon dried marjoram

1 cup sweet corn kernels (thawed if using frozen, drained if using canned)

1. In a large stockpot or Dutch oven, heat the olive oil over medium-high heat until glistening. Add the scallops, sear on each side, and cook until opaque, 60 to 90 seconds. Remove from the heat and set aside.

2. Add the onion, potatoes, and celery and cook for about 5 minutes, uncovered, stirring occasionally to prevent sticking. Add the oysters, bay leaves, and broth and bring to a boil. Reduce the heat and simmer for 10 minutes, or until the potatoes are tender.

3. In a measuring cup or bowl, combine the milk, white pepper, and marjoram and whisk together. Add the mixture to the stockpot along with the corn. Cook over medium heat for 5 to 10 minutes until the vegetables are cooked to your desired tenderness.

4. Return the seared scallops to the pot, heat through, and serve immediately.

Flavor boost: Typically, cooked bacon is used to add deep flavor to creamy chowders. Using smoked oysters creates a similar savory, umami-like flavor and offers an additional source of seafood nutrition in this recipe.

Per serving: Calories: 390; Fat: 19g; Protein: 38g; Cholesterol: 200mg; Sodium: 1370mg; Carbohydrates: 17g; Fiber: 2g

Gulf Coast Seafood Stew

SERVES 6 | PREP TIME 15 MINUTES | **COOK TIME** 1 HOUR

Nothing goes to waste when making this soup. Use leftover vegetable ends and shrimp peels to add extra flavor to stocks and broths. The longer cooking time adds a satisfying depth of flavor, but if you're short on time, you can skip this step and rely on chicken or vegetable broth instead. Creole seasoning adds the warming southern comfort of this Gulf classic.

GLUTEN-FREE,
DAIRY-FREE

1½ pounds unpeeled,
   medium raw shrimp

2 celery stalks, ends
   reserved and chopped

1 large yellow onion, peel
   reserved and chopped

8 cups Chicken Broth
   (page 24)

12 ounces Andouille sausage,
   cut into ½-inch slices

1 tablespoon olive oil

1 green bell pepper, chopped

3 garlic cloves, minced

1 pound red potatoes,
   halved or quartered

1 tablespoon fresh thyme (or
   ½ tablespoon dried thyme)

2 bay leaves

2 teaspoons Creole
   seasoning, such as Old Bay

1 pound fresh white fish fillets
   (such as cod, snapper,
   or haddock), cubed

½ pound cooked crawfish tails

Black pepper

1. Peel the shrimp and place the shrimp peels and tails in a stockpot. (Return the shrimp to the refrigerator until ready to use.) Add the celery ends and onion peel, then add the broth. Bring to a boil over medium-high heat, then reduce the heat and simmer for 30 minutes.

2. Combine the olive oil, onion, celery, sausage, and bell pepper in a separate large stockpot or Dutch oven and sauté on medium-high heat until the onion is translucent, 5 to 7 minutes. Add the garlic and sauté for 1 minute until fragrant, then add the potatoes, thyme, bay leaves, and Creole seasoning. Stir to combine.

3. Use a strainer to remove the shrimp peels and other solids from the broth mixture. Add the vegetable and sausage mixture to the broth and bring to a simmer. Cook 15 to 20 minutes or until the potatoes are fully tender.

4. Add the fish and shrimp and cook 2 to 3 minutes until the shrimp become pink and fish is opaque. Add the crawfish tails and heat through. Season with pepper to taste, then remove from the heat. Serve immediately.

Recipe tip: Look for cooked crawfish tails in the frozen seafood section of your grocery store. However, if you cannot find them, feel free to substitute additional shrimp, fish, or your other favorite type of seafood instead.

Per serving: Calories: 360; Fat: 11g; Protein: 25g; Cholesterol: 80mg; Sodium: 590mg; Carbohydrates: 42g; Fiber: 3g

Quick Cod Stew

SERVES 8 | **PREP TIME** 15 MINUTES | **COOK TIME** 30 MINUTES

Trying to incorporate more seafood into your diet? Research shows eating seafood two to three times per week reduces the risk of death from any health-related cause. For this stew, select a firm fish like cod which will stand up to the heat of the flavorful broth.

DAIRY-FREE

2 tablespoons olive oil

1 large onion, chopped

2 green bell peppers, chopped

6 garlic cloves, minced

1 teaspoon dried oregano

1 teaspoon dried thyme

1 (14.5-ounce) can crushed tomatoes

1 tablespoon tomato paste

1 (8-ounce) bottle clam juice

2 cups Classic Vegetable Broth (page 22)

1 tablespoon Worcestershire sauce

2 pounds cod, cut into 2-inch pieces

Salt

Black pepper

Hot sauce, optional

Chopped fresh parsley, for garnish

1. In a large wide pot or Dutch oven, heat the olive oil over medium-high heat. Add the onion and bell peppers and sauté until the onion is translucent and the vegetables are tender, 5 to 7 minutes. Add the garlic and sauté until fragrant, 1 to 2 minutes.

2. Add the oregano and thyme. Stir to combine with the vegetables. Reduce the heat to medium-low, add the tomatoes and tomato paste, and cook for 10 minutes.

3. Add the clam juice, broth, Worcestershire sauce, and cod. Bring to a simmer and cook until the fish is cooked through and flakes apart, 3 to 5 minutes.

4. Season with salt and pepper to taste. Add hot sauce, if using. Garnish with parsley.

Flavor boost: Looking to add a touch of creaminess? Stir in ½ cup of coconut milk.

Substitution tip: Any firm white fish will work well in this recipe. Sub in halibut, red snapper, or sea bass.

Per serving: Calories: 360; Fat: 11g; Protein: 25g; Cholesterol: 80mg; Sodium: 590mg; Carbohydrates: 42g; Fiber: 3g

Maryland-Style Crab Soup

SERVES 8 | PREP TIME 15 MINUTES | **COOK TIME** 55 MINUTES

Maryland crab soup is a vegetable-based crab soup instead of a cream-based soup. It's an East Coast signature when it's crabbing season. Regardless of where you live, this recipe can be prepared using fresh or canned crab depending on cost and what is available.

DAIRY-FREE

2 tablespoons olive oil

1 medium onion, diced

2 medium carrots, peeled and diced

1 medium potato, diced

1 cup frozen sweet corn

1 cup frozen shelled edamame

1 cup frozen peas

½ tablespoon Creole seasoning, such as Old Bay

2 teaspoons mustard powder

1 (14.5-ounce) can petite diced tomatoes

2 tablespoons tomato paste

8 cups Classic Vegetable Broth (page 22)

2 tablespoons Worcestershire sauce

1½ pounds cooked crabmeat

Salt

Black pepper

¼ cup chopped fresh parsley

1. In a large pot, heat the olive oil over medium–high heat. Add the onion, carrots, and potato and sauté until the onion is translucent and the vegetables begin to become tender, 5 to 7 minutes. Add the corn, edamame, and peas. Stir in the Creole seasoning and mustard powder.

2. Add the tomatoes, tomato paste, broth, and Worcestershire sauce. Bring to a boil, then reduce to a simmer and cook for 25 to 30 minutes, until the vegetables are fork tender.

3. Stir in the crabmeat. Simmer for an additional 10 to 15 minutes.

4. Season with salt and pepper to taste. Garnish with the parsley.

Ingredient tip: Opt for jumbo lump crabmeat if possible. Be sure to pick through and discard any shells that may be buried inside.

Substitution tip: Replace crab with another seafood if you prefer, like shrimp, scallops, or lobster.

Per serving: Calories: 260; Fat: 6g; Protein: 23g; Cholesterol: 45mg; Sodium: 1470mg; Carbohydrates: 27g; Fiber: 6g

Egg Drop Soup with Crab

SERVES 8 | PREP TIME 10 MINUTES | **COOK TIME** 20 MINUTES

Add a twist to the classic egg drop soup (see page 37) with this new seafood-inspired variation. The addition of crab and peas elevates the classic to a comforting new recipe. There are many minerals and nutrients that can reduce inflammation throughout the body, including omega-3 fatty acids, copper, and selenium, all of which are found in crabmeat.

DAIRY-FREE, QUICK
PREP, FAST

8 cups Chicken Stock
(page 25)

1 tablespoon grated
fresh ginger

1 tablespoon low-
sodium soy sauce

1½ tablespoons cornstarch

3 large eggs

1 tablespoon toasted
sesame oil

Salt

Black pepper

2 (6-ounce) cans crabmeat,
preferably jumbo lump,
picked over (about 2 cups)

1 cup frozen peas

4 scallions, thinly
sliced, for garnish

1. In a large pot, bring the stock and ginger to a boil.

2. In a small bowl, whisk together the soy sauce and cornstarch until the cornstarch has dissolved. If more liquid is needed to dissolve the cornstarch, use a little of the broth. Add the soy sauce mixture to the stock and boil for an additional 1 to 2 minutes, until the soup has slightly thickened. Remove the pot from the heat.

3. In a medium bowl, whisk together the eggs, sesame oil, and salt and pepper to taste. Slowly pour the egg mixture into the hot broth, at the same time whisking the broth constantly to break up the eggs as they cook in the soup.

4. Add the crabmeat and peas. Cook until warmed through.

5. Season with additional salt and pepper to taste. Garnish with the scallions.

Ingredient tip: To grate ginger, use a Microplane.

Substitution tip: Arrowroot starch is a 1-to-1 easy swap for cornstarch in this recipe.

Substitution tip: To make this gluten-free, use a gluten-free soy sauce, like tamari.

Per serving: Calories: 180; Fat: 7g; Protein: 15g; Cholesterol: 105mg; Sodium: 660mg; Carbohydrates: 13g; Fiber: <1g

Fisherman's Stew

SERVES 8 | PREP TIME 20 MINUTES | **COOK TIME** 50 MINUTES

Fisherman's stew, also known as cioppino, is considered by many to be the signature dish of San Francisco. Back in the 1800s, Italian immigrant fishermen would share the day's catch with other fishermen who came home empty-handed. The stew is a grab bag of ingredients and can easily be adapted to what's available. Don't rush the simmering process, which allows for all the flavors to develop.

DAIRY-FREE,
GLUTEN-FREE

2 tablespoons olive oil

1 large onion, diced

2 fennel bulbs, cored
  and diced

5 garlic cloves, minced

1 teaspoon fennel seeds

½ teaspoon dried oregano

½ teaspoon red
  pepper flakes

1 (28-ounce) can
  crushed tomatoes

6 cups Classic Vegetable
  Broth (page 22)

1 (8-ounce) bottle clam juice

½ pound cod, cut into
  2-inch pieces

1 pound large shrimp,
  shelled and deveined

1 pound bay scallops

12 littleneck clams, scrubbed

12 mussels, scrubbed

Salt

Black pepper

¼ cup minced fresh
  parsley, for garnish

1. In a large wide pot or Dutch oven, heat the olive oil over medium-high heat. Add the onion and fennel and sauté until the onion is translucent and the vegetables are tender, 5 to 7 minutes. Stir in the garlic, fennel seeds, oregano, and red pepper flakes and cook until fragrant, 1 to 2 minutes.

2. Add the tomatoes, broth, and clam juice. Bring to a boil, then reduce to a simmer and cook for 30 minutes.

3. Add the seafood one at a time, evenly dispersing them throughout the pot: cod, shrimp, scallops, clams, and mussels. Reduce the heat to a simmer. Cover and cook until the seafood is cooked through and shellfish open, about 10 minutes. (Discard any mussels that have not opened.)

4. Season with salt and pepper to taste. Garnish with the parsley.

Substitution tip: Load up on the seafood you enjoy the most and use less of or remove what you don't.

Per serving: Calories: 210; Fat: 4g; Protein: 24g; Cholesterol: 100mg; Sodium: 1100mg; Carbohydrates: 19g; Fiber: 5g

Thai-Style Shrimp Noodle Soup

SERVES 8 | **PREP TIME** 15 MINUTES | **COOK TIME** 35 MINUTES

This easy soup makes a healthy meal that is perfect for lunch or dinner. Made with succulent shrimp, creamy coconut milk, fragrant Thai red curry spices, broth, veggies, and rice noodles, it highlights how heat, spice, and flavor can make nourishing ingredients exciting to enjoy.

DAIRY-FREE,
GLUTEN-FREE

14 ounces rice noodles

1 tablespoon coconut oil

5 garlic cloves, minced

3 tablespoons minced
    fresh ginger

Zest and juice of
    1 lime, divided

2 lemongrass stalks,
    thinly sliced

¼ cup red curry paste

8 cups Classic Vegetable
    Broth (page 22)

5 makrut lime leaves, sliced
    down the middle vertically

3 tablespoons fish sauce

2 (14-ounce) cans light
    coconut milk

4 baby bok choy, sliced

1½ pounds shrimp,
    shelled and deveined

½ cup chopped fresh cilantro

Salt

Black pepper

1. Cook the rice noodles according to package directions, then set aside.

2. In a large pot, heat the coconut oil over medium-high heat. Add the garlic, ginger, lime zest, and lemongrass. Sauté for 2 minutes or until fragrant, being careful not to burn the garlic. Stir in the red curry paste to coat the vegetables.

3. Add the broth, lime leaves, and fish sauce. Bring to a simmer and cook for 15 minutes.

4. Add the coconut milk and bok choy and simmer for 5 minutes. Add the shrimp and continue to simmer until the shrimp is cooked through and no longer pink, 3 to 4 minutes.

5. Remove from the heat and stir in the rice noodles, lime juice, and cilantro.

6. Season with salt and pepper to taste.

Flavor boost: Makrut lime leaves are responsible for the distinctive lime-lemon aroma and flavor that are an indispensable part of Thai cuisine. Cutting them allows the flavor to develop stronger in the broth.

Flavor boost: Adjust the level of spice by increasing or decreasing the amount of red curry paste, to suit your taste.

Per serving: Calories: 280; Fat: 9g; Protein: 15g; Cholesterol: 105mg; Sodium: 1460mg; Carbohydrates: 30g; Fiber: 2g

Coconut Curry Soup with Shrimp

SERVES 8 | **PREP TIME** 15 MINUTES | **COOK TIME** 25 MINUTES

Skip takeout and make this simple coconut curry soup with shrimp at home. It is bursting with delicious flavor and tastes just like it came from a Thai restaurant. Canned coconut milk usually has a thick, cream-like consistency. It is higher in fat, and people typically use it for baking or cooking.

DAIRY-FREE

2 tablespoons coconut oil

2 shallots, finely chopped

2 red bell peppers, thinly sliced

2 cups thinly sliced cremini mushrooms

4 garlic cloves, minced

1 tablespoon minced fresh ginger

3 tablespoons red curry paste

8 cups Chicken Stock (page 25)

3 tablespoons low-sodium soy sauce

3 teaspoons fish sauce

2 (14-ounce) cans light coconut milk

2 pounds large shrimp, shelled and deveined

Juice of 1 lime

¼ cup chopped scallions

¼ cup chopped Thai basil

Salt

Black pepper

1. In a large pot, heat the coconut oil over medium-high heat. Add the shallots, bell peppers, and mushrooms, and sauté until the vegetables are tender, 5 to 7 minutes. Add the garlic and ginger. Sauté until fragrant, 1 to 2 minutes. Add the red curry paste and stir to coat the vegetables.

2. Add the stock, soy sauce, fish sauce, and coconut milk. Bring to a simmer.

3. Add the shrimp and cook until they turn pink, 3 to 5 minutes.

4. Remove from the heat and stir in the lime juice, scallions, and Thai basil.

5. Season with salt and pepper to taste.

Ingredient tip: Make sure to slice vegetables thin for every bite to melt in your mouth.

Substitution tip: Can't find Thai basil? Use twice the amount of regular basil as a substitution.

Per serving: Calories: 270; Fat: 11g; Protein: 24g; Cholesterol: 150mg; Sodium: 1530mg; Carbohydrates: 10g; Fiber: 2g

Cajun Shrimp Gumbo

SERVES 6 | PREP TIME 10 MINUTES | **COOK TIME** 45 MINUTES

Gumbo is year-round comfort food: It's savory, spicy, warm, and filling, and since you can adjust the heat level, it can be modified to fit anyone's tastes. This version features freekeh, a fluffy, rice-like whole grain that adds additional nutrients and fiber.

DAIRY-FREE,
QUICK PREP

¼ cup olive oil

¼ cup all-purpose flour

1 large yellow onion, chopped

3 green bell peppers, chopped

2 garlic cloves, minced

1 (14.5-ounce) can diced tomatoes, with juices

1½ cups Chicken Stock (page 25)

1 tablespoon chili powder

½ tablespoon smoked paprika

½ teaspoon dried oregano

1 bay leaf

⅛ teaspoon cayenne pepper

1. Create a roux by heating the olive oil in a stockpot or Dutch oven. Add the flour and whisk together. Continue cooking, scraping the sides of the pan, until the roux becomes a dark caramel color, about 20 minutes.

2. Add the onion, bell peppers, garlic, and tomatoes and stir to combine. Cook until the onion becomes translucent, about 5 minutes. Add the stock, chili powder, paprika, oregano, bay leaf, cayenne pepper, salt, and pepper and bring to a low simmer over high heat.

3. Reduce to low heat and add the shrimp and okra. Stir to combine and adjust the heat to maintain a simmer. Add the kale, allowing it to wilt and combine.

4. Ladle the gumbo into bowls and top with the freekeh. Serve immediately.

Recipe tip: Freekeh is an ancient grain that originated in Africa. It's a version of cracked wheat, so be sure to note that it is not gluten-free, though many other ancient grains are. If using a grain substitute, be sure to adjust cooking time accordingly.

Salt

Black pepper

1½ pounds shrimp,
   peeled and deveined

1 cup frozen okra (do
   not defrost)

2 cups shredded kale

2 cups cooked freekeh

Ingredient tip: To cook freekeh: Use a 2.5-to-1 ratio of liquid to grain. Using the same method as quinoa or rice, bring the liquid to a boil, add the uncooked grains, and simmer until all liquid is absorbed. If prepping in large batches, allow to cool before transferring to the refrigerator.

Ingredient tip: Okra often has the reputation of being slimy, but this can be avoided by using frozen okra. Do not rinse your frozen okra, simply pat dry and add directly to the simmering gumbo. Any sliminess that is released will serve to further thicken the stew.

Per serving: Calories: 380; Fat: 12g; Protein: 25g; Cholesterol: 145mg; Sodium: 960mg; Carbohydrates: 43g; Fiber: 9g

Shrimp Boil in a Bowl

SERVES 6 | PREP TIME 10 MINUTES | **COOK TIME** 30 MINUTES

This speedy version of a classic Cajun shrimp boil fest takes little time to prepare, but pays off with big flavor. Shrimp boils often include crawfish as well, but for simplicity they are omitted here. Serve as is or add a scoop of cooked white rice gumbo-style.

DAIRY-FREE, FAST,
GLUTEN-FREE,
QUICK PREP

1 tablespoon olive oil

9 ounces Andouille sausage,
   cut into ½-inch slices

1 small yellow onion,
   chopped

1½ cups sweet corn kernels

1 teaspoon Old Bay
   seasoning

5 cups Chicken Broth
   (page 24) or seafood broth

3 cups quartered red
   potatoes (skin on)

1 pound medium
   shrimp, peeled

Lemon wedges, for serving

1. Heat the olive oil in a large stockpot or Dutch oven over medium-high heat. Add the sausage and onion and sauté until the sausage begins to brown, about 4 minutes. Add the corn and sauté 2 to 3 minutes more. Add the Old Bay seasoning and stir to combine.

2. Add the broth and bring to a boil. Add the potatoes, then reduce the heat and simmer, uncovered, 10 to 15 minutes, until the potatoes are fully tender.

3. Remove from the heat, then add the shrimp and place the lid on top. Allow to sit 3 to 4 minutes to cook the shrimp, then adjust the seasoning as needed. Ladle into bowls and serve with lemon wedges.

Substitution tip: If you are sensitive to spice or sodium, replace the andouille sausage with mild kielbasa sausage or additional shrimp. Note that Old Bay seasoning can be very high in sodium, so swap for a low-sodium Creole seasoning if desired.

Per serving: Calories: 320; Fat: 16g; Protein: 22g; Cholesterol: 120mg; Sodium: 1010mg; Carbohydrates: 25g; Fiber: 2g

Simple Korean Kimchi Jjigae with Shrimp

SERVES 4 | PREP TIME 10 MINUTES | **COOK TIME** 30 MINUTES

Jjigae refers to a Korean style stew and many variations exist. This version using kimchi is among the most popular, and for good reason. It's simple to prepare at home, so don't let the idea of cooking a Korean dish intimidate you! If desired, serve with a side of white or brown rice (not included in the nutritional analysis).

DAIRY-FREE,
GLUTEN-FREE,
QUICK PREP

1 tablespoon sesame oil

1 small onion, thinly sliced

3 garlic cloves, thinly sliced

1 pound kimchi, with juices

1 teaspoon salt

2 teaspoons sugar

1 tablespoon Korean
   chili flakes

1 tablespoon gochujang
   (Korean red pepper paste)

3 cups Chicken Broth
   (page 24)

1 (14-ounce) package firm
   tofu, drained and cut
   into ¼-inch slices

1 pound medium shrimp,
   peeled and thawed,
   if using frozen

1 teaspoon sesame oil

1 scallion, thinly sliced

1. In a large stockpot, heat the sesame oil over medium-high heat. Add the onion and garlic, and cook for about 5 minutes, until the onion starts to soften.

2. Add the kimchi and sauté for 2 minutes. Then add the salt, sugar, chili flakes, gochujang, and broth. Stir until combined. Bring to a simmer, cover, and cook for 10 minutes.

3. Uncover and lay the sliced tofu over the top. Replace the cover and simmer for another 10 minutes. Uncover, then add the shrimp and stir in the sesame oil. Garnish with the scallion and serve immediately.

Ingredient tip: Korean chili flakes tend to be milder, so if using a full tablespoon seems like too much or if you need to substitute for a different type of chili flake, be sure to adjust the seasoning appropriately for your tastes.

Per serving (without rice): Calories: 330; Fat: 15g; Protein: 36g; Cholesterol: 145mg; Sodium: 1630mg; Carbohydrates: 16g; Fiber: 5g

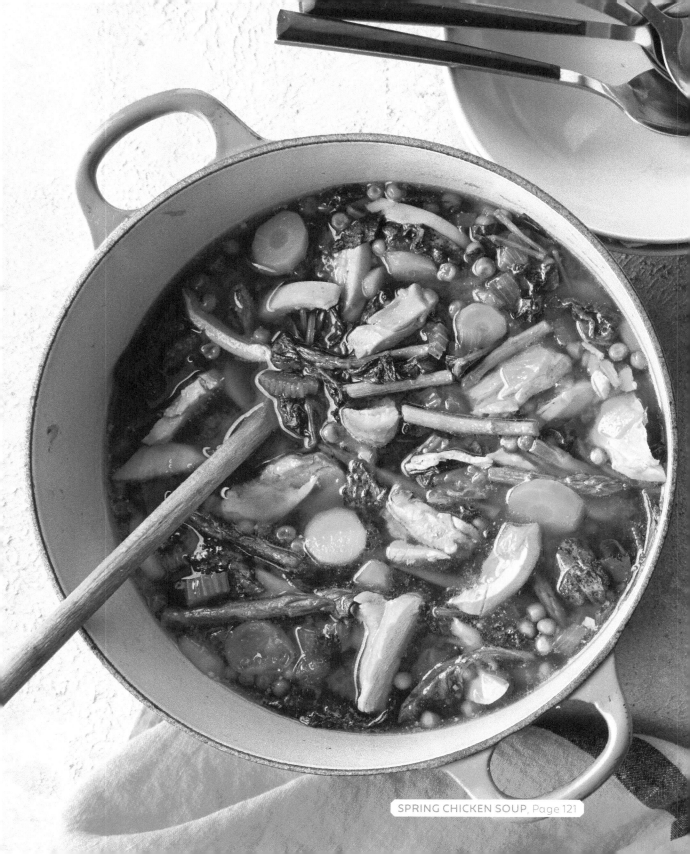

SPRING CHICKEN SOUP, Page 121

7

Poultry Soups

C hicken noodle soup is the quintessential recipe that we turn to when we are looking for some warming comfort. Poultry soups go way beyond the classic chicken noodle soup, though, and we took that concept and ran with it! This chapter is full of nourishing recipes inspired by global cuisines. Looking to save time? Pick up a precooked rotisserie chicken and let it serve double-duty: Shred the meat to use in one of these soups, and save the bones to create a flavorful chicken broth (see page 24).

Chicken Zoodle Soup

SERVES 6 | PREP TIME 15 MINUTES | **COOK TIME** 30 MINUTES

Chicken zoodle soup is similar to the classic chicken noodle soup (see page 34), but packed with a big boost of anti-inflammatory vegetables. Zucchini is high in water and contains significant amounts of fiber, electrolytes, and other nutrients that are necessary for a healthy digestive system.

GLUTEN-FREE,
DAIRY-FREE

2 tablespoons olive oil

1 medium onion, diced

3 medium carrots,
    peeled and diced

2 celery stalks, diced

4 garlic cloves, minced

½ teaspoon dried thyme

½ teaspoon dried rosemary

½ teaspoon dried basil

1 bay leaf

6 cups Chicken Stock
    (page 25)

3 large zucchini, spiralized

2 cups chopped
    cooked chicken

2 tablespoons lemon juice

Salt

Black pepper

1. In a large pot, heat the olive oil over medium-high heat. Add the onion, carrots, and celery and sauté until the onion is translucent and the vegetables are tender, 5 to 7 minutes. Add the garlic and cook until fragrant, 1 to 2 minutes.

2. Add the thyme, rosemary, basil, and bay leaf. Stir the herbs to coat the vegetables.

3. Add the stock. Bring to a boil, then reduce to a simmer and cook for 10 minutes.

4. Add the zucchini and chicken, continuing to simmer the soup until the zucchini is tender and the chicken is warmed through.

5. Stir in the lemon juice. Season with salt and pepper to taste.

Ingredient tip: Don't have a spiralizer? Most grocery stores now carry vegetable noodles in their produce or frozen sections.

Flavor boost: Acidity in a soup can really make a difference. Add the lemon juice at the end of cooking to maximize its bright flavor.

Per serving: Calories: 260; Fat: 11g; Protein: 20g; Cholesterol: 40mg; Sodium: 460mg; Carbohydrates: 20g; Fiber: 4g

Miso Chicken Noodle Soup

SERVES 6 | **PREP TIME** 10 MINUTES | **COOK TIME** 20 MINUTES

Start with the miso soup recipe (see page 30) in chapter 2 and enhance it with a few additional ingredients to create this next-level miso chicken noodle soup. Packed with protein coming from both the chicken and edamame, this comforting soup will leave you full and satisfied. Cut the mushrooms thin to match the delicate broth.

DAIRY-FREE, FAST,
GLUTEN-FREE,
QUICK PREP

1 tablespoon sesame oil

1 cup thinly sliced
 mushrooms

2 scallions, chopped

3 garlic cloves, minced

6 cups Miso Soup (page 30)

1 cup water

2 ounces rice noodles

1½ cups shredded
 cooked chicken

1 cup frozen shelled
 edamame

Salt

Black pepper

1. In a large pot, heat the sesame oil over medium-high heat. Add the mushrooms and sauté until tender, 8 to 10 minutes. Stir in the scallions and garlic. Sauté for an additional 1 to 2 minutes.

2. Add the miso soup and water. Bring to a boil, then reduce to a simmer.

3. Add the rice noodles, chicken, and edamame and simmer for 5 minutes, until noodles are tender.

4. Season with salt and pepper to taste.

Ingredient tip: Make miso soup ahead of time and store in the refrigerator up to 4 days.

Ingredient tip: You can regrow scallions by saving the white ends. Simply place them in a small cup of water, and as they begin to sprout, replant them in a pot.

Per serving: Calories: 210; Fat: 8g; Protein: 17g; Cholesterol: 25mg; Sodium: 540mg; Carbohydrates: 16g; Fiber: 5g

Lemon Chicken Orzo Soup

SERVES 8 | PREP TIME 10 MINUTES | **COOK TIME** 25 MINUTES

Tender chicken is complemented by a vibrant lemony broth and orzo pasta. Lemons are high in heart-healthy vitamin C and several beneficial plant compounds that can help lower cholesterol.

FAST, DAIRY-FREE, QUICK PREP

2 tablespoons olive oil

1 large onion, diced

3 medium carrots, peeled and diced

5 garlic cloves, minced

2 tablespoons chopped fresh rosemary

1 lemon, zested and sliced, divided

6 cups Chicken Stock (page 25)

2 cups water

2 bay leaves

¾ cup whole-wheat orzo pasta

2 cups shredded cooked chicken breast

Salt

Black pepper

2 tablespoons chopped fresh parsley

1. In a large stockpot, heat the olive oil over medium-high heat. Add the onion and carrots and sauté until the onion is translucent and the vegetables are tender, 5 to 7 minutes. Add the garlic and sauté until fragrant, 1 to 2 minutes.

2. Add the rosemary and lemon zest. Stir to coat the vegetables.

3. Add the lemon slices, stock, water, and bay leaves. Bring to a boil. Stir in the orzo and chicken. Reduce the heat to a simmer and cook until orzo is tender, 10 to 12 minutes.

4. Remove bay leaves. Season with salt and pepper to taste. Garnish with the parsley.

Flavor boost: Use citrus zest in recipes to provide lemon flavor without the acidity from the juice.

Per serving: Calories: 230; Fat: 8g; Protein: 16g; Cholesterol: 30mg; Sodium: 320mg; Carbohydrates: 24g; Fiber: 4g

Spring Chicken Soup

SERVES 6 | PREP TIME 10 MINUTES | **COOK TIME** 30 MINUTES

The phrase "spring chicken" evokes a sense of energetic youth with some bounce in your step. We can't guarantee that's what this soup will do for you, but it is chock-full of some of the best spring produce. If you're cooking it later in the year, use frozen or canned produce in place of ingredients that aren't at the peak of freshness.

DAIRY-FREE,
GLUTEN-FREE,
QUICK PREP

2 tablespoons olive oil

1 large onion, diced

1 large carrot, sliced

2 celery stalks, sliced

2 garlic cloves, minced

Salt

Black pepper

4 boneless, skinless chicken
  thighs (about 1 pound)

2 medium parsnips,
  peeled and chopped

2 cups halved cherry
  tomatoes

6 cups Chicken Stock
  (page 25)

4 cups baby spinach

1 small bunch Swiss or
  rainbow chard, stemmed
  and chopped

1 cup green peas

10 thin spears asparagus,
  trimmed and cut
  to 1-inch pieces

1. In a large stockpot or Dutch oven, heat the olive oil over medium-high heat. Add the onion, carrot, and celery and sauté until the onion is translucent, about 5 minutes. Add the garlic and season with salt and pepper, then cook about 1 minute more.

2. Add the chicken, parsnips, and tomatoes, then cover with the stock. Bring to a boil, then reduce the heat and simmer, uncovered, for about 20 minutes.

3. Use a slotted spoon to remove the chicken thighs. Roughly chop the cooked chicken, then return to the pot. Add the spinach, Swiss chard, peas, and asparagus and simmer about 5 minutes more.

4. Season with salt and pepper to taste. Serve immediately.

Ingredient tip: Asparagus is a perennial favorite for the springtime but there is variability in the size of the stalks. The ends are woody and fibrous, so remove those before cooking, regardless of the thickness of each spear. If using thick spears, add to the pot earlier to allow them to cook to a crisp-tender texture. If using thinner spears, add them later in the cooking process.

Per serving: Calories: 310; Fat: 10g; Protein: 28g; Cholesterol: 60mg; Sodium: 600mg; Carbohydrates: 28g; Fiber: 6g

Turkey and Meatball Kale Soup

SERVES 6 | PREP TIME 30 MINUTES | **COOK TIME** 30 MINUTES

This soup offers fresh lemon flavor in every bite—in the broth as well as the meatballs. As the soup simmers, the flavors will continue to intensify.

DAIRY-FREE

For the meatballs

1 pound 93% lean
   ground turkey

5 garlic cloves, minced

¼ cup chopped fresh parsley

3 scallions, chopped

Zest of 1 lemon

¼ teaspoon salt

⅛ teaspoon black pepper

For the soup

2 tablespoons olive oil

2 shallots, minced

2 medium carrots,
   peeled and chopped

3 celery stalks, chopped

4 garlic cloves, minced

1 teaspoon ground cumin

⅛ teaspoon cayenne pepper

8 cups Chicken Broth
   (page 24)

To make the meatballs

1. Preheat the oven to 350°F. Line a baking sheet with parchment paper.

2. In a large bowl, combine the turkey, garlic, parsley, scallions, zest, salt, and pepper. Roll the mixture into small balls (about the size of a ping pong ball) and place on the prepared baking sheet.

3. Bake for 15 to 20 minutes, until the meatballs begin to brown and the internal temperature reaches 165°F.

To make the soup

1. In a large pot, heat the olive oil over medium-high heat. Add the shallots, carrots, and celery and sauté until the shallots are translucent and the vegetables are tender, 5 to 7 minutes. Add the garlic and sauté until fragrant, 1 to 2 minutes.

2. Add the cumin and cayenne pepper. Stir to coat the vegetables.

3. Add the broth and soy sauce. Add the lemon juice, then drop the remaining lemon into the broth to infuse more lemon flavor.

1 tablespoon low-sodium soy sauce

1 lemon, juiced, reserving pieces of lemon

3 cups chopped kale

Salt

Black pepper

4. Add the kale and continue to simmer until it has wilted.

5. Season with salt and pepper to taste.

Flavor boost: Want more heat? Add more cayenne pepper.

Flavor boost: The addition of lemon zest in the meatballs infuses a strong lemon flavor without the acidity.

Per serving: Calories: 260; Fat: 13g; Protein: 24g; Cholesterol: 55mg; Sodium: 430mg; Carbohydrates: 16g; Fiber: 3g

Leftover Thanksgiving Turkey Soup

SERVES 6 | PREP TIME 15 MINUTES | **COOK TIME** 40 MINUTES

Have a few mismatched ingredients leftover from preparing your holiday dinner? Utilize your leftovers to create a brand-new meal. This is a Thanksgiving Day meal all put together in a delicious bowl of soup.

DAIRY-FREE,
GLUTEN-FREE

2 tablespoons olive oil

1 large onion, chopped

2 large carrots, peeled
and chopped

3 celery stalks, chopped

4 garlic cloves, chopped

1 teaspoon dried thyme

1 tablespoon Italian
seasoning

½ pound green beans,
cut into 1-inch pieces

1 large sweet potato,
peeled and chopped

2 cups frozen corn

8 cups Chicken Stock
(page 25)

2 cups shredded
cooked turkey

Salt

Black pepper

1. In a large pot, heat the olive oil over medium-high heat. Add the onion, carrots, and celery and sauté until the onion is translucent and the vegetables are tender, 5 to 7 minutes. Add the garlic and sauté until fragrant, 1 to 2 minutes.

2. Add the thyme and Italian seasoning. Stir to coat the vegetables. Add the green beans, sweet potatoes, and corn.

3. Add the stock. Bring to a boil then reduce to a simmer. Simmer for 30 minutes, until the vegetables are tender. Stir in the turkey.

4. Season with salt and pepper to taste.

Ingredient tip: Don't let your Thanksgiving turkey carcass go to waste! Save the bones and create a rich and flavorful turkey broth or stock. Follow the same directions for the chicken stock (see page 25) and replace with turkey bones.

Per serving: Calories: 300; Fat: 10g; Protein: 22g; Cholesterol: 50mg; Sodium: 590mg; Carbohydrates: 30g; Fiber: 4g

Greek Lemon Chicken Soup

SERVES 6 | PREP TIME 5 MINUTES | **COOK TIME** 20 MINUTES

Classically known as avgolemono, this soup gets its name from the Greek words for egg and lemon. *Utilize your culinary skills to gently temper the eggs in the hot broth. Since this is a very simple recipe with only six ingredients, the quality of the chicken broth matters. Use a very flavorful chicken broth and whip this soup together in about 20 minutes.*

DAIRY-FREE, FAST,
QUICK PREP

10 cups Chicken
  Broth (page 24)

1 cup orzo pasta

4 large eggs

⅔ cup fresh lemon juice

3 cups shredded
  cooked chicken

3 cups baby spinach

Salt

Black pepper

1. In a large pot, bring the broth to a boil. Reduce to a brisk simmer, add the orzo, and cover the pot. Cook until the orzo is al dente, about 10 minutes.

2. As the orzo is cooking, in a medium bowl, whisk the eggs and lemon juice.

3. When the orzo is cooked, ladle about 1 cup of the hot broth slowly into the egg mixture, whisking constantly. (This process tempers the eggs, so you don't end up with scrambled eggs in your soup.) Set aside.

4. Stir in the chicken and baby spinach and cook until the spinach has wilted. Reduce the heat to medium-low. Stir the egg mixture into the soup and let cook for 2 to 3 minutes, until the broth has slightly thickened.

5. Season with salt and pepper to taste.

Culinary term: In cooking, tempering is a technique used when combining two ingredients of radically different temperatures. Do this step slowly so they both gradually rise to the same temperature and the quality of the ingredients stays unchanged.

Per serving: Calories: 370; Fat: 10g; Protein: 38g; Cholesterol: 185mg; Sodium: 260mg; Carbohydrates: 34g; Fiber: 4g

Stracciatella Soup with Chicken

SERVES 4 | **PREP TIME** 10 MINUTES | **COOK TIME** 15 MINUTES

Stracciatella is an Italian version of egg drop soup. Stracciatella means "little shred" in Italian, which perfectly describes the egg in this light, nourishing soup. The addition of chicken turns this classic into a hearty and filling meal.

FAST, GLUTEN-FREE,
QUICK PREP

8 cups Chicken Broth
(page 24)

4 large eggs

¼ cup finely grated
Parmesan cheese

¼ cup chopped fresh parsley

2 cups baby spinach

1 cup shredded
cooked chicken

Salt

Black pepper

1. In a large pot, bring the broth to a boil over medium-high heat.

2. In a bowl, whisk together the eggs, Parmesan cheese, and parsley.

3. Reduce the heat to medium-low to allow the broth to come down to a simmer. Stir the broth in a circular motion. Slowly pour the egg mixture into the moving broth, stirring gently to create thin egg ribbons.

4. Stir in the spinach and chicken.

5. Season with salt and pepper to taste.

Flavor boost: The key to this soup is starting with a flavorful broth as this is a simplistic recipe with few ingredients. Refer to chapter 2 for our broth and stock recipes.

Recipe tip: For the classic version, omit the chicken.

Per serving: Calories: 240; Fat: 11g; Protein: 30g; Cholesterol: 220mg; Sodium: 390mg; Carbohydrates: 7g; Fiber: 0g

Red Italian Wedding Soup

SERVES 8 | **PREP TIME** 30 MINUTES | **COOK TIME** 50 MINUTES

The tomato-based variation to the classic Italian wedding soup (see page 38) doesn't get the attention it deserves. The tomato-based broth has a hint of sweetness that is balanced with the savory meatballs.

For the meatballs

1 pound 93% lean
  ground turkey

½ cup whole-wheat
  bread crumbs

1 egg, beaten

2 tablespoons grated
  Parmesan cheese

1 tablespoon garlic powder

½ tablespoon fennel seeds

1 tablespoon Italian
  seasoning

½ teaspoon salt

¼ teaspoon black pepper

To make the meatballs

1. Preheat the oven to 400°F. Line a baking sheet with parchment paper.

2. In a large bowl, combine the turkey, bread crumbs, egg, Parmesan cheese, garlic powder, fennel seeds, Italian seasoning, salt, and pepper. Mix well to combine.

3. Shape the mixture into ½-inch meatballs and place on the prepared baking sheet. Bake for 15 to 20 minutes, until the internal temperature reaches 165°F. Remove from the oven and set aside.

To make the soup

1. In a large stockpot, heat the olive oil over medium-high heat. Add the onion, carrots, and celery and sauté until the onion is translucent and the vegetables are tender, 5 to 7 minutes. Add the garlic and sauté until fragrant, 1 to 2 minutes.

2. Add the broth, water, tomatoes, tomato paste, vinegar, Italian seasoning, and red pepper flakes; stir to combine. Bring to a boil, then reduce to a simmer and cook for 20 minutes.

Continued

For the soup

2 tablespoons olive oil

1 medium onion, chopped

3 medium carrots,
    peeled and chopped

2 celery stalks, chopped

3 garlic cloves, minced

6 cups Chicken Broth
    (page 24)

1½ cups water

1 (28-ounce) can
    crushed tomatoes

2 tablespoons tomato paste

2 teaspoons balsamic
    vinegar

1 tablespoon Italian
    seasoning

½ teaspoon red
    pepper flakes

3 cups chopped
    baby spinach

1 cup cooked whole-wheat
    orzo pasta

Salt

Black pepper

3. Add the meatballs and simmer for an additional 10 minutes, until the meatballs warm through and soak up the soup flavors.

4. Add the spinach and orzo and cook until the spinach has wilted.

5. Season with salt and pepper to taste.

Flavor boost: Balance a sweet tomato-based brothy soup with a hit of acidity. The addition of balsamic vinegar can help balance the flavors of the broth base.

Storage tip: Meal prepping these meatballs in advance can help complete this recipe in a shorter amount of time. The beauty of meatballs is that you can freeze them either at the uncooked or cooked stage. According to the USDA, uncooked ground meat is freezer-safe for up to 3 to 4 months, and cooked ground meat is safe for 2 to 3 months.

Per serving: Calories: 310; Fat: 11g; Protein: 22g; Cholesterol: 65mg; Sodium: 440mg; Carbohydrates: 34g; Fiber: 7g

Chicken Tortilla Soup

SERVES 8 | PREP TIME 10 MINUTES | **COOK TIME** 25 MINUTES

Just like some of the other classic soups in this cookbook, there are many versions of chicken tortilla soup. Our version is simmered to perfection with vegetables, beans, corn, tomatoes, and chicken. Plus, you have many options for mix and match toppings to create a new version every time. This strategy works particularly well when prepping large batches because you'll avoid the rut of boredom. Combine new toppings or spices to create a unique meal experience even when enjoying leftovers. This comforting soup is ready in just 35 minutes.

GLUTEN-FREE,
QUICK PREP

2 tablespoons olive oil

1 large onion, diced

1 jalapeño, seeded and
   finely chopped

1 small zucchini, chopped

4 garlic cloves, chopped

1 teaspoon dried oregano

1 teaspoon chili powder

1 teaspoon ground cumin

3 cups Chicken Stock (page 25)

1 cup water

2 (14.5-ounce) cans fire-
   roasted diced tomatoes

Juice of 1 lime

1. In a large stockpot, heat the olive oil over medium-high heat. Add the onion, jalapeño, and zucchini and sauté until the onion is translucent and the vegetables are tender, 5 to 7 minutes.

2. Add the garlic and sauté until fragrant, 1 to 2 minutes.

3. Add the oregano, chili powder, and cumin. Stir to coat the vegetables.

4. Add the stock, water, diced tomatoes, and lime juice. Bring to a boil, then reduce to a simmer.

5. Add the black beans, cannellini beans, corn, and chicken. Simmer for 15 minutes.

6. Season with salt and pepper to taste. Add toppings as desired.

Continued

1 (15-ounce) can black beans, drained and rinsed

1 (15-ounce) can cannellini beans, drained and rinsed

1 cup frozen corn

2 cups shredded cooked chicken breast

Salt

Black pepper

Diced avocado, plain Greek yogurt, chopped cilantro, tortilla chips, for topping (optional)

Ingredient tip: Look for low-sodium or no-salt-added canned beans. Always drain and rinse the beans to remove more sodium before adding them to recipes.

Per serving: Calories: 280; Fat: 6g; Protein: 22g; Cholesterol: 30mg; Sodium: 510mg; Carbohydrates: 35g; Fiber: 8g

Thai Chicken Soup with Lemongrass

SERVES 6 | **PREP TIME** 10 MINUTES | **COOK TIME** 25 MINUTES

This flavorful soup features some of the signature flavors in Thai cuisine. If you live in a warm climate or are able to source makrut lime leaves, they can be a unique ingredient to cook with. If they're not available, sub in fresh lime juice instead.

DAIRY-FREE,
GLUTEN-FREE,
QUICK PREP

1 tablespoon coconut oil

1 shallot, minced

1 Thai chili or serrano pepper,
  seeded and minced

1 tablespoon grated
  fresh ginger

2 garlic cloves, minced

2½ tablespoons yellow or
  sweet curry powder

4 cups Chicken Stock
  (page 25)

3 makrut lime leaves
  (or 2 tablespoons
  fresh lime juice and
  1 teaspoon lime zest)

1 (13.5-ounce) can light
  coconut milk

1. Heat the coconut oil in a large stockpot or Dutch oven over medium-high heat. Add the shallot and sauté 3 minutes or until soft. Add the chili, ginger, and garlic and sauté until fragrant, about 1 minute more. Add the curry powder and stir to combine.

2. Add the stock, lime leaves, and coconut milk. Gently crush the lemongrass to release the aromatics and add to the pot. Stir to combine and bring to a simmer. Cook, uncovered, for 15 to 20 minutes.

3. After the flavors have combined, stir in the carrots, scallions, and chicken and return to a simmer. Cook until the chicken is heated through.

4. Ladle the soup into bowls, removing the lemongrass. Serve with the cilantro, pepper, and a lime wedge.

Continued

2 (2-inch) pieces
   lemongrass, peeled

1 large carrot, sliced
   thin or grated

3 scallions, thinly sliced

2 cups shredded
   cooked chicken

1 cup chopped fresh cilantro

Black pepper

Fresh lime wedges,
   for serving

Flavor boost: Look for curry powder blends that are deep orange in color. These often list turmeric as one of the first ingredients. The curcumin compound in turmeric is more bioavailable when paired with the pepperin compound in black pepper, so don't forget the pepper grinder when you serve this soup.

Per serving: Calories: 220; Fat: 12g; Protein: 17g; Cholesterol: 40mg; Sodium: 300mg; Carbohydrates: 11g; Fiber: 2g

White Chicken Chili

SERVES 8 | **PREP TIME** 15 MINUTES | **COOK TIME** 30 MINUTES

This chili is made with hearty beans, tender chicken, and a rich and creamy broth with zero dairy. Using mashed beans lends this soup creaminess. It is a culinary technique you can also use to thicken sauces.

DAIRY-FREE,
GLUTEN-FREE

2 tablespoons olive oil

1 large onion, diced

1 jalapeño pepper, seeded
and finely diced

4 garlic cloves, minced

1 (7-ounce) can green chiles

1 tablespoon ground cumin

1 teaspoon dried oregano

¼ teaspoon red
pepper flakes

2 (15-ounce) cans cannellini
beans, drained and
rinsed, divided

6 cups Chicken Broth
(page 24)

Juice of 1 lime

4 cups shredded
cooked chicken

Salt

Black pepper

½ cup chopped fresh cilantro

1. In a large pot, heat the olive oil over medium-high heat. Add the onion and jalapeño and cook until the onion is translucent and the vegetables are tender, 5 to 7 minutes. Add the garlic and cook until fragrant, 1 to 2 minutes.

2. Add the green chiles, cumin, oregano, and red pepper flakes. Stir to combine.

3. In a blender or food processor, add 1 cup of the beans with ¼ cup of the broth. Blend until smooth and creamy.

4. Add the blended bean mixture, the remaining 5½ cups of broth, and lime juice to pot. Bring to a gentle boil and cook for 10 minutes. Add the remaining whole beans and chicken. Reduce to a simmer and cook for an additional 5 minutes until the chicken and beans warm through.

5. Season with salt and pepper to taste. Garnish with cilantro.

Flavor boost: Canned green chiles come with different spice levels. Choose the spice level that you would enjoy best!

Per serving: Calories: 310; Fat: 7g; Protein: 34g; Cholesterol: 60mg; Sodium: 500mg; Carbohydrates: 29g; Fiber: 6g

Chipotle Turkey Chili

SERVES 8 | PREP TIME 10 MINUTES | **COOK TIME** 45 MINUTES

This turkey chili is just as hearty and filling as a traditional chili. With ours, you'll notice the addition of extra veggies, but feel free to make swaps and substitutions for ingredients as desired. The bulk of the flavor comes from the chipotle chile in adobo sauce.

DAIRY-FREE,
GLUTEN-FREE,
QUICK PREP

1 tablespoon olive oil

1 pound 93% lean
   ground turkey

1 green bell pepper, chopped

1 large yellow onion,
   chopped

3 celery stalks, chopped

2 (15-ounce) cans chili
   beans, with juices

2 (14.5-ounce) cans
   diced chili-style
   tomatoes, with juices

1 (6-ounce) can tomato paste

1½ cups Chicken
   Broth (page 24)

1 chipotle chile in adobo
   sauce, finely diced

2 garlic cloves, minced

1½ teaspoons ground cumin

¼ teaspoon black pepper

Fresh cilantro, for garnish

1. Heat the olive oil in a large heavy-bottomed pot over medium-high heat and stir in the turkey. Brown until the turkey is fully cooked and no longer pink, 5 to 7 minutes. Transfer the cooked turkey to a dish or bowl and set aside.

2. Return the pot to medium-high heat and add the bell pepper, onion, and celery. Cook until the vegetables are tender, 5 to 6 minutes.

3. Stir in the chili beans, tomatoes, tomato paste, broth, chipotle, garlic, cumin, and pepper. Stir to combine, then add the cooked turkey back to the pot. Simmer 30 minutes, covered, stirring occasionally. Serve immediately with cilantro.

Ingredient tip: There are many vegetables that would work well in this chili recipe. To cut down on food waste, use what you have on hand, including other colors of bell pepper, chopped kale or spinach, or thinly sliced carrots.

Flavor boost: Chipotle chiles in adobo sauce can pack a punch. If you prefer less heat, select a smaller pepper or omit the sauce. If you want it spicier, you can always add more. Freeze chipotle chile leftovers from the can in an ice cube tray and preserve for later use.

Per serving: Calories: 330; Fat: 10g; Protein: 25g; Cholesterol: 55mg; Sodium: 850mg; Carbohydrates: 36g; Fiber: 9g

Roasted Poblano and White Bean Chicken Chili

SERVES 6 | **PREP TIME** 10 MINUTES | **COOK TIME** 1 HOUR

Although this is a relatively quick-cooking chili, the flavors will continue to blend and build the longer you extend the cooking time. If you're in a hurry, this stovetop version can be done in less than an hour, but if you have time to spare, consider simmering the ingredients longer. See below for notes on a slow cooker version.

GLUTEN-FREE,
QUICK PREP

2 tablespoons olive oil

1 yellow onion, diced

1 large poblano pepper,
   seeded and diced

Salt

Black pepper

3 garlic cloves, minced

1 tablespoon ground cumin

1 tablespoon ground
   coriander

1½ teaspoons chili powder

1½ teaspoons smoked
   paprika

⅛ teaspoon liquid
   smoke (optional)

4 cups Chicken Stock
   (page 25)

Juice and zest of 1 small lime

1. Heat the olive oil in a large stockpot or Dutch oven over medium-high heat. Add the onion, poblano pepper, salt, and pepper and sauté for 5 to 7 minutes or until softened.

2. Add the garlic, cumin, coriander, chili powder, paprika, and liquid smoke, if using, and sauté 1 minute more. Add the stock, scraping the bottom of the pot with a wooden spoon to deglaze it.

3. Bring the soup to a boil, then reduce to a simmer. Add the lime juice and zest, corn, beans, and chicken. Cook 30 to 45 minutes, stirring occasionally.

4. To serve, ladle the chili into bowls and top with the cilantro, avocado, and sour cream.

Continued

1 cup sweet corn kernels,
    thawed if using frozen

2 (15-ounce) cans Great
    Northern beans,
    drained and rinsed

2 large chicken breasts,
    cooked and shredded

½ cup chopped fresh cilantro

1 avocado, diced

½ cup sour cream

Slow cooker option: Add all ingredients except the cilantro, avocado, and sour cream to the bowl of your slow cooker. Cook on high for 4 hours or low for 6 hours. Stir to combine and adjust seasoning as needed. To serve, top with fresh cilantro, avocado, and sour cream.

Per serving: Calories: 430; Fat: 16g; Protein: 26g; Cholesterol: 40mg; Sodium: 320mg; Carbohydrates: 49g; Fiber: 11g

Chimichurri Chicken and Rice Soup

SERVES 4 | **PREP TIME** 15 MINUTES | **COOK TIME** 30 MINUTES

This simple soup lets the chimichurri sauce take center stage. Chimichurri is a traditional South American condiment that is often paired with seafood, beef, or potatoes. It adds freshness and acidity to the broth of this chicken and rice soup. Try leftover chimichurri as a fun topper for other recipes.

GLUTEN-FREE

For the chimichurri

½ cup chopped fresh parsley

¼ cup chopped
    fresh oregano

½ cup diced red onion

4 garlic cloves, peeled

¼ cup red wine vinegar

½ cup olive oil

½ tablespoon red
    pepper flakes

¼ teaspoon salt

⅛ teaspoon black pepper

To make the chimichurri

In a food processor, combine the parsley, oregano, onion, garlic, vinegar, olive oil, red pepper flakes, salt, and pepper. Pulse several times until combined, leaving some chunks in the mixture. Transfer to a small bowl to allow flavors to combine, then set aside until ready to use.

To make the soup

1. Heat the olive oil in a large stockpot or Dutch oven over medium-high heat. Add the carrots, celery and onion, and sauté until the onion is translucent, about 5 minutes.

2. Add the scallions, chicken, chimichurri, stock, and rice. Season with salt and pepper to taste.

3. Bring to a simmer and cook, partially covered, until the rice is tender, about 20 minutes. Add the milk, then cook 5 minutes more.

4. To serve, ladle the soup into serving bowls and top with 1 tablespoon of chimichurri sauce. Serve immediately.

Continued

For the soup

2 tablespoons olive oil

2 large carrots, sliced

1 celery stalk, sliced

1 small yellow onion, diced

2 scallions, thinly sliced

1 pound boneless chicken
    breast, cubed

⅓ cup chimichurri sauce,
    plus more for garnish

4 cups Chicken Stock
    (page 25)

1 cup brown or wild rice

1 cup milk

Storage tip: You will have more chimichurri sauce than is needed for this recipe. To store, place in an airtight container. Use within 1 to 2 days if leaving at room temperature, or place in the refrigerator. Remove prior to re-serving and allow the oil to warm to room temperature and return to a liquid consistency.

To use a slow cooker: Place all ingredients except for the milk into your slow cooker. Cook on high for 4 hours or low for 6 hours. Fold in the milk and stir to combine. Garnish with additional chimichurri sauce before serving.

Per serving: Calories: 340; Fat: 11g; Protein: 25g; Cholesterol: 65mg; Sodium: 310mg; Carbohydrates: 36g; Fiber: 2g

For the chimichurri only (1 tablespoon)

Per serving: Calories: 50; Fat: 5g; Protein: 0g; Cholesterol: 0mg; Sodium: 30mg; Carbohydrates: 1g; Fiber: 0g

Stuffed Pepper Stew

SERVES 8 | **PREP TIME** 15 MINUTES | **COOK TIME** 45 MINUTES

Make dinnertime even easier and turn time-consuming stuffed peppers into a simple one-pot meal. This soup deconstructs a traditional stuffed pepper recipe and contains all the same ingredients. Capsanthin, found in red bell peppers, is a powerful antioxidant responsible for their brilliant color.

DAIRY-FREE

2 tablespoons olive oil

1 large onion, diced

4 garlic cloves, minced

2 pounds 93% lean ground turkey

1 tablespoon Italian seasoning

6 cups Chicken Stock (page 25)

1 (14.5-ounce) can crushed tomatoes

1 (28-ounce) can fire-roasted diced tomatoes, with juices

2 red bell peppers, chopped

1 green bell pepper, chopped

1 tablespoon Worcestershire sauce

1½ cups cooked brown rice

Salt

Black pepper

¼ cup chopped fresh parsley

1. In a large pot, heat the olive oil over medium-high heat. Add the onion and sauté until it is translucent and tender, 5 to 7 minutes. Add the garlic and cook until fragrant, 1 to 2 minutes. Add the turkey, breaking it up into small pieces. Continue to cook until no pink remains, 5 to 7 minutes. Drain any excess fat.

2. Stir in the Italian seasoning, stock, crushed tomatoes, diced tomatoes, red and green bell peppers, and Worcestershire sauce. Bring to a simmer and cook for 25 to 30 minutes, until the peppers are tender.

3. Stir in the rice.

4. Season with salt and pepper to taste. Garnish with the parsley.

Ingredient tip: Did you know? Bell peppers with three bumps at the bottom are considered "male" peppers and are less sweet, but their seeds stay intact at the top. Bell peppers with four bumps are considered "female" peppers and are subtly sweeter and their seeds tend to fall down into the cavity of the pepper.

Per serving: Calories: 230; Fat: 9g; Protein: 18g; Cholesterol: 45mg; Sodium: 720mg; Carbohydrates: 21g; Fiber: 3g

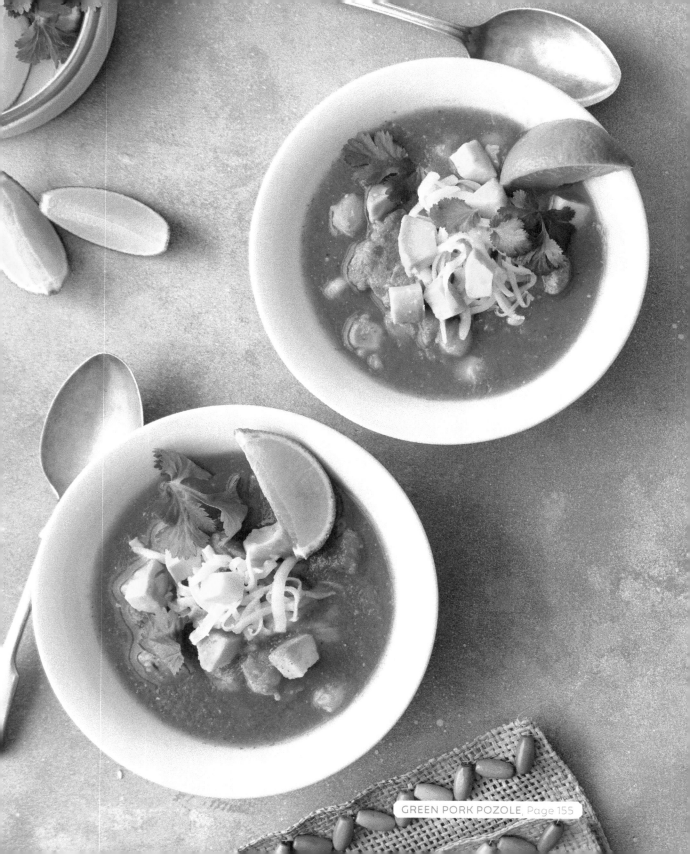

GREEN PORK POZOLE, Page 155

8

Meaty Soups and Stews

Meat contains a valuable amount of protein and key nutrients, like zinc and vitamin B12 to maintain a healthy immune system. While these nutrients may also be sourced from plant-based foods, meat can still be part of vegetable-forward eating if you enjoy the taste and texture. Opt for lean meat like beef, bison, pork, lamb, and oxtail, which are featured in this chapter. The delicious soups and stews in this section are also chock-full of vegetables, legumes, herbs, and spices that align with an anti-inflammatory diet.

Chili Mac

SERVES 8 | PREP TIME 10 MINUTES | **COOK TIME** 20 MINUTES

This hearty Midwestern fare shows up in a variety of forms depending on regional and family preferences. Our version is thicker, similar to goulash. If you prefer a thinner consistency, simply add water, ½ cup at a time, until you reach your desired thickness. This soup provides fiber from two types of beans, plus lycopene from the diced tomatoes.

FAST, QUICK PREP

1 tablespoon olive oil

1 small onion, diced

2 garlic cloves, minced

1 pound 93% lean
   ground beef

4 cups Chicken Broth
   (page 24)

1 (28-ounce) can
   diced tomatoes

2 teaspoons chili powder

1½ teaspoons ground cumin

Salt

Black pepper

10 ounces uncooked
   elbow or rotini pasta

1 (15-ounce) can black beans,
   drained and rinsed

1 (15-ounce) can kidney
   beans, drained and rinsed

1 cup shredded
   cheddar cheese

2 tablespoons chopped
   fresh parsley or cilantro

Up to 2 cups water (optional)

1. Heat the olive oil in a large skillet or Dutch oven over medium-high heat. Add the onions, garlic, and beef and cook until browned, about 5 minutes.

2. Stir in the broth, tomatoes, chili powder, and cumin. Season with salt and pepper to taste. Quickly bring to a simmer and add the pasta. Bring to a boil, then reduce the heat and cover. Cook until the pasta is tender, 10 to 12 minutes.

3. Remove from the heat. Add the black and kidney beans, carefully folding them in until evenly combined. Top with the cheddar cheese, then cover and allow to sit for 2 to 3 minutes, or until the cheese melts.

4. Garnish with the parsley. Serve immediately.

Ingredient tip: Swap ground beef for lean ground turkey if desired.

Flavor boost: If you enjoy more spice, try adding crushed red pepper flakes or chopped or sliced jalapeños.

Per serving: Calories: 440; Fat: 10g; Protein: 21g; Cholesterol: 20mg; Sodium: 380mg; Carbohydrates: 69g; Fiber: 8g

Beef and Barley Soup

SERVES 8 | **PREP TIME** 20 MINUTES | **COOK TIME** 1 HOUR 10 MINUTES

Loaded with nutritious veggies, tender beef, and plump barley, this soup is a complete meal in a bowl! One of the most notable benefits of including beef in your diet is its ability to build and maintain muscle. As we age, getting the right amount of protein becomes increasingly important to fight off diseases.

DAIRY-FREE

½ cup all-purpose flour

1 teaspoon salt

1 teaspoon black pepper

1 pound boneless beef chuck roast, fat trimmed off and cubed

2 tablespoons olive oil

1 large onion, chopped

2 large carrots, peeled and chopped

2 celery stalks, chopped

4 garlic cloves, minced

2 teaspoons dried oregano

½ cup red wine

3 tablespoons tomato paste

4 cups Beef Stock (page 26)

1. In a shallow dish combine the flour, salt, and pepper. Dredge the beef cubes with flour, shaking off the excess.

2. Heat the olive oil in a Dutch oven or large stockpot over medium-high heat. Add the beef and cook, turning to brown the meat on all sides. Do this in two or three batches, so as not to crowd the pot. Remove the meat from the pot and set aside.

3. In the same pot, add the onion, carrots, celery, garlic, and oregano. Cook the vegetables until soft, 5 to 7 minutes, stirring occasionally.

4. Add the wine, scraping the bottom to deglaze it. Let simmer and reduce the wine by half. Add the tomato paste and stir to coat the vegetables.

5. Add the beef back to the pot along with the stock and water. Stir to combine.

Continued

4 cups water

¾ cup hulless barley

4 cups baby spinach

1 tablespoon chopped
fresh parsley

6. Bring to a boil, add the barley, and turn down to a simmer for 45 to 50 minutes, until the meat is tender and the barley is cooked through. Stir occasionally so the barley doesn't stick together. If you find that too much liquid has evaporated or the soup is too thick, add more water as necessary until you get the desired consistency.

7. Remove the soup from the heat and stir in the spinach until it wilts. Season with salt and pepper as needed. Garnish with the parsley.

Flavor boost: Why brown the beef? The caramelization of the meat lends rich flavor to the finished dish. And meat dredged in flour before browning adds body to the sauce.

Ingredient tip: Just one 3-ounce serving of cooked beef provides 10 essential nutrients, including protein, zinc, iron, and B vitamins.

Per serving: Calories: 240; Fat: 6g; Protein: 18g; Cholesterol: 35mg; Sodium: 610mg; Carbohydrates: 25g; Fiber: 5g

Beef and Mushroom Stew

SERVES 8 | **PREP TIME** 15 MINUTES | **COOK TIME** 1 HOUR 45 MINUTES

This simple beef and mushroom stew comes together quickly then braises slowly to a flavorful finish. Mushrooms are a type of fungus that have a uniquely savory flavor known as umami and a dense, meaty texture when cooked.

DAIRY-FREE

2 tablespoons olive oil

2 pounds boneless
   beef chuck roast, cut
   into 1-inch cubes

¼ teaspoon salt

¼ teaspoon black pepper

1 pound cremini
   mushrooms, sliced

2 medium onions, sliced

4 garlic cloves, minced

1 cup red wine

4 cups Beef Stock (page 26)

1 tablespoon tomato paste

½ teaspoon dried parsley

½ teaspoon dried rosemary

½ teaspoon dried sage

½ teaspoon dried thyme

2 tablespoons flour

2 tablespoons water

1. Preheat the oven to 325°F.

2. In an ovenproof wide pot or Dutch oven, heat the olive oil over medium-high heat. Season the beef with the salt and pepper, then add the beef, in batches if necessary, and brown. Remove the beef from the pot with a slotted spoon and set aside.

3. Add mushrooms and onions to the pot and sauté until tender, 7 to 10 minutes. Add the garlic and cook until fragrant, 1 to 2 minutes. Add the wine, scraping any bits off the bottom to deglaze it.

4. Stir in the stock, tomato paste, parsley, rosemary, sage, and thyme. Return the beef to the pot. Bring to a boil. Cover and bake for 1 hour.

5. In a small bowl, whisk together the flour and water. Remove the stew from the oven, then stir in the slurry. Cover and cook for another 30 minutes, until the stew is thick and the beef is tender.

6. Season with salt and pepper to taste.

Substitution tip: Replace the red wine with additional beef stock, if desired.

Continued

Recipe tip: Chuck roast is your best bet for beef stew, but it's also a pretty tough cut so it needs time to break down and become tender. Rush the cooking process and the beef will be tough and chewy. Cooking it low and slow yields tender beef.

Per serving: Calories: 370; Fat: 9g; Protein: 42g; Cholesterol: 75mg; Sodium: 430mg; Carbohydrates: 32g; Fiber: 4g

Cabbage Roll Soup

SERVES 8 | **PREP TIME** 15 MINUTES | **COOK TIME** 40 MINUTES

This unstuffed cabbage roll soup has all the same flavor as classic baked cabbage rolls, but with much less work! Cabbage, an inexpensive vegetable available year-round, contains glutamine, which has been noted to strengthen the immune system.

DAIRY-FREE,
GLUTEN-FREE

1 tablespoon olive oil

1 large onion, diced

3 garlic cloves, minced

1 pound 93% lean
ground beef

4 cups chopped
green cabbage

2 large carrots peeled,
quartered, and sliced

4 cups Beef Stock (page 26)

2 (15-ounce) cans
crushed tomatoes

½ cup brown rice

1 bay leaf

2 tablespoons brown sugar

Salt

Black pepper

2 tablespoons chopped
fresh parsley

1. In a large pot, heat the olive oil over medium-high heat. Add the onion and sauté until it is translucent, about 5 minutes. Add the garlic and cook until fragrant, 1 to 2 minutes.

2. Add the beef and break it up into small pieces with a wooden spoon. Cook until the beef is browned, 4 to 5 minutes.

3. Add the cabbage, carrots, stock, tomatoes, rice, bay leaf, and brown sugar. Bring to a simmer and cook for 25 minutes, until the rice is tender. Remove the bay leaf and discard.

4. Season with salt and pepper to taste. Top with parsley.

Ingredient tip: Ground beef that is 93 percent lean or leaner meets government guidelines for "lean" and is an excellent choice if you want a meat option. It works well in dishes that require crumbles, like meat sauce, tacos, soups, or stuffed peppers, where draining fat might be difficult.

Per serving: Calories: 250; Fat: 8g; Protein: 17g; Cholesterol: 35g; Sodium: 510mg; Carbohydrates: 28g; Fiber: 4g

Ginger Couscous Meatball Soup

SERVES 6 | PREP TIME 20 MINUTES | **COOK TIME** 30 MINUTES

Ginger is pungent and spicy with a very slight woody flavor. This particular ingredient is as aromatic as it is flavorful. With ginger in the meatballs and simmering in the broth, this soup is vibrant, fresh, and delicious.

DAIRY-FREE

For the meatballs

1 pound 93% lean
   ground beef

¼ cup sliced scallions

1 tablespoon grated
   fresh ginger

2 garlic cloves, minced

1 tablespoon low-
   sodium soy sauce

½ tablespoon ground cumin

⅛ teaspoon cayenne pepper

¼ teaspoon salt

⅛ teaspoon black pepper

To make the meatballs

1. Preheat the oven to 400°F. Line a baking sheet with parchment paper.

2. In a medium bowl, mix together the beef, scallions, ginger, garlic, soy sauce, cumin, cayenne pepper, salt, and pepper. Shape the mixture into ½-inch meatballs and place on the prepared baking sheet. Bake for 15 to 20 minutes, until the internal temperature reaches 165°F. Remove from the oven and set aside.

To make the soup

1. In a large pot, heat the olive oil over medium-high heat. Add the onion and sauté for 5 minutes, until it is translucent. Add the garlic and ginger and sauté until fragrant, 1 to 2 minutes. Add the mushrooms and cook for another 5 minutes until the moisture of the mushrooms is released and evaporated.

2. Add the broth and soy sauce. Stir to combine. Bring to a boil.

For the soup

1 tablespoon olive oil

1 medium onion, diced

4 garlic cloves, minced

2 teaspoons minced
 fresh ginger

2 cups sliced cremini
 mushrooms

8 cups Mushroom
 Broth (page 29)

1 tablespoon low-
 sodium soy sauce

½ cup Israeli couscous

1 tablespoon sesame seeds

3. Turn the soup down to a simmer, add the meatballs and couscous and cover. Cook until the couscous is tender, 10 to 15 minutes.

4. Serve and top with sesame seeds.

Ingredient tip: Ginger is knobby with many bumps and grooves. Instead of using a vegetable peeler, use a spoon to peel the skin off of ginger.

Per serving: Calories: 230; Fat: 11g; Protein: 21g; Cholesterol: 50g; Sodium: 960mg; Carbohydrates: 14g; Fiber: 2g

Easy Beef Pho

SERVES 6 | PREP TIME 15 MINUTES | **COOK TIME** 40 MINUTES

If you love pho and always wanted to give it a try at home, I think you'll be surprised how straightforward it actually is! This is a quick, satisfying, and full-flavor version of Vietnam's national dish. You'll be slurping up noodles in just 45 minutes.

DAIRY-FREE,
GLUTEN-FREE

For the broth

1 tablespoon olive oil

1 large onion, chopped

1 (2-inch) piece fresh ginger, peeled and sliced

3 cinnamon sticks

8 cups Beef Stock (page 26)

4 cups water

1 tablespoon star anise (about 6)

½ tablespoon whole cloves

¼ cup fish sauce

2 teaspoons sugar

For the pho

12 ounces rice noodles

1 small onion, thinly sliced

1 pound sirloin, sliced thin

5 scallions, sliced thin on a bias

2 cups bean sprouts

1 mint bunch, stemmed

1 basil bunch, stemmed

1 cilantro bunch, stemmed

2 jalapeños, sliced thin

2 limes, sliced into wedges

To make the broth

In a large pot, heat the olive oil over medium heat. Add the onion, ginger, and cinnamon sticks. Cook for 3 to 5 minutes, stirring occasionally. Add the stock, water, star anise, cloves, fish sauce, and sugar. Stir, lower the heat to a gentle simmer, and cook for 20 minutes.

To make the pho

1. Meanwhile, cover the rice noodles with hot water and soak for 8 minutes (or follow the instructions on the package). Drain and set aside.

2. Discard the onion, ginger, cinnamon sticks, star anise, and cloves from the broth.

3. In six bowls, evenly divide the rice noodles, onion, sirloin, scallions, bean sprouts, mint, basil, cilantro, and jalapeños. Pour the hot broth over the pho. (The hot broth will cook the sirloin.) Serve immediately.

Ingredient tip: Putting the steak in the freezer 45 to 60 minutes prior to cutting makes it easier to slice.

Flavor boost: The star anise pod is shaped like a star (hence its name). It has a very strong, distinct flavor that is sweet and spicy, similar to licorice.

Per serving: Calories: 410; Fat: 6g; Protein: 29g; Cholesterol: 45mg; Sodium: 1730mg; Carbohydrates: 58g; Fiber: 3g

Sweet Potato Chili

SERVES 8 | PREP TIME 15 MINUTES **| COOK TIME** 50 MINUTES

Sweet potato chili is a healthy and quick dinner recipe that is full of lean bison, black beans, corn, and lots of flavor! The tender sweet potatoes are rich in antioxidants that prevent free radical damage and are an excellent source of beta-carotene, which can be converted to vitamin A and help support your immune system and gut health.

GLUTEN-FREE

2 tablespoons olive oil

1 medium onion, chopped

1 pound ground bison

1 teaspoon chili powder

2 teaspoons ground cumin

1 teaspoon smoked paprika

⅛ teaspoon ground
    cinnamon

4 cups cubed peeled
    sweet potatoes

1 (28-ounce) can
    crushed tomatoes

1 cup Beef Stock (page 26)

1 (15-ounce) can sweet whole
    kernel corn, drained

1 (15-ounce) can black beans,
    drained and rinsed

Salt

Black pepper

Greek yogurt, salsa,
    chopped cilantro, for
    topping (optional)

1. In a large pot, heat the olive oil over medium-high heat. Add the onion and sauté until it is translucent, about 5 minutes. Add the bison and cook, breaking it up into pieces, until browned. Drain any excess fat.

2. Add the chili powder, cumin, paprika, and cinnamon; stir to combine.

3. Add the sweet potatoes, tomatoes, and stock; stir to combine. Bring to a simmer, cover, and cook for 20 to 25 minutes.

4. Add the corn and black beans; stir to combine. Cover and simmer for 10 to 15 minutes, until the sweet potatoes are tender.

5. Season with salt and pepper to taste. Add toppings, if using.

Substitution tip: Can't find ground bison? Use ground beef or turkey instead.

Ingredient tip: When choosing canned vegetables or beans, look for a low-sodium or no-salt-added option.

Per serving: Calories: 280; Fat: 8g; Protein: 19g; Cholesterol: 30mg; Sodium: 470mg; Carbohydrates: 37g; Fiber: 9g

Russian Borscht

SERVES 6 | PREP TIME 10 MINUTES | **COOK TIME** 1 HOUR 30 MINUTES

Borscht is actually a Ukrainian recipe, but it is very popular in Russia as well as communities across the US. It differs from a vegetable-based soup because the veggies are sautéed separately, instead of cooking in the broth itself. If stew meat isn't available, you can also use ground beef in its place.

GLUTEN-FREE,
QUICK PREP

1 tablespoon olive oil

1 pound beef stew meat,
    trimmed and cut
    into small cubes

6 cups Beef Stock (page 26)

2 large carrots, peeled

2 large beets, peeled

1 large russet potato, peeled

2 celery stalks, sliced thin

8 ounces shredded green
    cabbage (about ¼
    medium cabbage head)

2 garlic cloves, minced

¼ cup tomato paste

1 tablespoon white vinegar

Salt

Pepper

¼ cup fresh parsley or
    dill, for garnish

1 cup sour cream, for garnish

1. Heat the olive oil over medium-high heat in a heavy-bottomed nonstick skillet. Add the stew meat and brown on all sides, about 5 minutes. Meanwhile, in a large stockpot or Dutch oven, bring the stock to a low simmer.

2. Once the beef is browned, transfer to the stock and simmer, stirring occasionally, for 1 hour.

3. In the meantime, shred the carrots, beets, and potato. Add the shredded vegetables, celery, and cabbage to the skillet, scraping the bottom of the pan to combine the flavors from browning the beef. Sauté for 15 minutes, until all the vegetables appear wilted and softened. Add the garlic and tomato paste. Transfer 1 cup of the hot stock to the skillet and simmer 3 to 5 minutes.

4. Stir in the vinegar, then carefully transfer the borscht to the stockpot with the beef. Season with salt and pepper to taste, then serve in bowls garnished with fresh parsley. Top with sour cream.

Substitution tip: If using ground beef, brown according to instructions. Once browned, follow step 2, but reduce simmering time to 20 to 25 minutes.

Per serving: Calories: 330; Fat: 14g; Protein: 25g; Cholesterol: 70mg; Sodium: 670mg; Carbohydrates: 28g; Fiber: 5g

Sausage, White Bean, and Escarole Soup

SERVES 6 | PREP TIME 10 MINUTES | **COOK TIME** 45 MINUTES

The classic combination of spicy sausage, creamy white cannellini beans, and bright escarole has never been so satisfying. Escarole is also one of the most fiber-rich greens in the produce aisle. A two-cup serving of raw escarole provides almost 10 percent of the daily value of vitamin A, which is essential for eye health, immune function, and cell growth. Cooking the escarole in this soup, concentrates the vitamin so you get a big dose with each serving.

GLUTEN-FREE, QUICK PREP

1 tablespoon olive oil

6 Italian sausage links, casings removed

1 medium onion, chopped

5 garlic cloves, minced

½ teaspoon crushed red pepper

1 large escarole head, chopped (about 6-8 cups)

½ cup dry white wine

2 (15-ounce) cans cannellini beans, drained and rinsed

2 cups Chicken Stock (page 25)

Salt

Black pepper

Grated Parmesan cheese, for garnish

1. In a large stockpot or Dutch oven, heat the olive oil over medium-high heat. Working in batches, add the sausage and sauté until it is cooked through, breaking it up with a spoon, about 6 minutes per batch. Using a slotted spoon, transfer the sausage to a dish lined with paper towels, leaving the drippings in the pot.

2. Reduce the heat to medium, add the onion, and sauté until it is translucent, 5 minutes. Add the garlic and cook until fragrant, 1 to 2 minutes. Mix in the crushed red pepper.

3. Add the escarole and sauté until wilted. Add the wine to the pot and scrape to deglaze the bottom.

4. Add the beans, stock, and cooked sausage. Bring the soup to a simmer and cook for 10 minutes.

5. Season with salt and pepper to taste. Garnish with Parmesan cheese.

Substitution tip: Looking for a leaner option? Try using Italian chicken sausage.

Continued

Flavor boost: Escarole looks a lot like a head of lettuce, but really it's a part of the chicory family, which also includes radicchio and endive. Chicories are closely related to lettuce, but they have a heartier texture and a bitter edge. The flavor is slightly nutty, with a balance of bitter and sweet.

Per serving: Calories: 640; Fat: 39g; Protein: 30g; Cholesterol: 90mg; Sodium: 990mg; Carbohydrates: 39g; Fiber: 10g

Green Pork Pozole

SERVES 6 to 8 | **PREP TIME** 15 MINUTES | **COOK TIME** 45 MINUTES

Pozole means "hominy," a key feature of this type of soup. There are other variations that use a red sauce or white sauce, but this green version includes tomatillos, fresh herbs, heart-healthy avocado, and two types of peppers. If you prefer more spice, add a jalapeño to the mix or include the seeds from your peppers to give it an extra kick.

GLUTEN-FREE

2 tablespoons olive oil

1 pound pork
tenderloin, cubed

Salt

Black pepper

1 pound fresh tomatillos,
husked and rinsed

1 large yellow onion, roughly
chopped or quartered

3 garlic cloves, peeled

2 poblano peppers,
seeded and chopped

1 serrano pepper, seeded
and chopped

1 small cilantro bunch,
chopped (about ¾ cup)

¼ cup loosely packed
fresh oregano leaves

1. Heat the olive oil in a large nonstick or cast iron skillet over medium-high heat. Season the pork with salt and pepper, then add the pork to the skillet and sear on all sides, about 5 minutes. Transfer to a plate or bowl to keep warm.

2. Meanwhile, place the tomatillos, onion, garlic, poblano and serrano peppers, cilantro, and oregano in a high-speed blender. Blend until smooth. Add the mixture to the heated skillet and cook, stirring occasionally, until the color darkens. Remove from the heat.

3. Add the stock to a large stockpot or Dutch oven and bring to a low simmer. Add the seared pork and cook 15 minutes, partially covered. Transfer the tomatillo sauce to the stockpot, then add the hominy. Stir to combine and return to a simmer. Adjust the seasoning if needed.

4. To serve, ladle into bowls and top with the cheese, avocado, and lime wedges.

Continued

8 cups Chicken Stock
(page 25)

2 (15-ounce) cans white
hominy, drained
and rinsed

1 cup shredded Monterey
jack cheese

1 avocado, diced

1 lime, cut into wedges,
for garnish

Substitution tip: Traditionally, there are many options for topping a pozole-style soup. Other suggestions include shredded lettuce or cabbage, thinly sliced radishes, minced onions, or sour cream or crema. This is another great option for using leftover veggies before they go to waste, so get creative!

Per serving: Calories: 420; Fat: 18g; Protein: 32g; Cholesterol: 75mg; Sodium: 880mg; Carbohydrates: 33g; Fiber: 6g

Slow-Cooker Cider-Spiced Pork Stew

SERVES 6 | PREP TIME 20 MINUTES | **COOK TIME** 3 to 4 HOURS ON HIGH OR 5 to 6 HOURS ON LOW

Although the combination of pork, mustard, and apples might seem an unexpected trio at first, you'll be convinced to add this slow-cooker soup into your regular rotation as soon as you lift the cover and smell the amazing aroma. The long, slow-cooking method allows the tartness and acidity of the apples and mustard to soften and blend together. Apple juice can serve as a substitute for apple cider if you prepare this recipe when seasonal apple cider is difficult to find.

DAIRY-FREE, FREEZER FRIENDLY

3 tablespoons canola or vegetable oil, divided

1½ pounds boneless pork shoulder, cut into 1½-inch cubes

1 teaspoon salt

½ teaspoon black pepper

1 large yellow onion, chopped

⅓ cup all-purpose flour

1 cup apple cider

4 cups Chicken Broth (page 24)

1½ tablespoons whole-grain mustard

2 teaspoons dried thyme

2 teaspoons dried sage

1 teaspoon dried oregano

½ pound small red potatoes, halved or quartered

1. Heat 2 tablespoons of canola oil over medium-high heat in a large heavy-bottomed skillet. Season the pork with the salt and pepper. Once the oil is heated, work in batches to sear the pork on all sides until browned, about 5 minutes per batch. Repeat until all the pork is seared, then transfer to a large slow cooker.

2. Add the remaining 1 tablespoon of canola oil to the skillet. Add the onion and cook 2 to 3 minutes, until it is softened. Stir in the flour and cook 2 minutes more. Add the apple cider to the skillet and deglaze the bottom with a wooden spoon. Whisk in the broth and mustard and bring to a boil. Once the mixture is boiling, remove it from the heat.

3. Add the thyme, sage, oregano, potatoes, carrots, and apple to the slow cooker. Carefully pour the hot broth mixture over the top. Place the lid of the slow cooker on top, then cook 5 to 6 hours on low, or 3 to 4 hours on high.

4. Stir to combine, then ladle into bowls and serve immediately.

Continued

4 carrots, peeled and
  sliced into ¼-inch coins

1 large apple (Granny Smith
  or Golden Delicious),
  cored and chopped

Storage tip: This is a freezer-friendly stew that can be stored up to 3 months. Portion individual servings or freeze in a larger batch. To thaw, transfer the frozen soup to the refrigerator overnight to defrost. Reheat in the microwave or on the stovetop once fully thawed to a liquid consistency in the refrigerator.

Per serving: Calories: 420; Fat: 22g; Protein: 25g; Cholesterol: 70mg; Sodium: 650mg; Carbohydrates: 30g; Fiber: 4g

Pork and Poblano Stew

SERVES 6 to 8 | **PREP TIME** 20 MINUTES | **COOK TIME** 1 HOUR 15 MINUTES

The charred flavor of the poblano peppers mixes well with the smoky spice of the adobo sauce and adds rich, deep flavor when allowed to cook slowly on the stovetop. This pork and poblano stew works with pork tenderloin as well, so feel free to swap for another cut of meat that suits your budget and preference.

GLUTEN-FREE, FREEZER FRIENDLY

4 large poblano peppers

2 tablespoons olive oil, divided

1½ pounds pork shoulder, trimmed and cubed

Salt

Black pepper

1 medium onion, chopped

1 teaspoon ground cumin

3 garlic cloves, minced

1 chipotle chile in adobo sauce, chopped

4 cups Chicken Stock (page 25)

1 tablespoon dried oregano

1 large sweet potato, peeled and chopped in ½-inch cubes

1½ cups sweet corn kernels (thawed if using frozen)

1. Set the oven's broiler to high. Brush the poblano peppers with 1 tablespoon of olive oil and place on a sheet pan lined with parchment paper. Broil, turning every 1 to 2 minutes, until the peppers are blackened and charred. Place in a mixing bowl and cover with foil. Allow them to rest and cool for 10 minutes, then remove the charred skin. It should easily peel away from the peppers. Slice them to remove the seeds and cut away the stems. Roughly chop and set aside.

2. Heat the remaining 1 tablespoon of olive oil in a large stockpot or Dutch oven over medium-high heat. Season the pork with salt and pepper. Working in batches to avoid overcrowding, add the pork to the pot and sear on all sides, about 5 minutes per batch. Continue until all the pork has been evenly seared. Once seared, set the pork aside.

3. In the same pot, add the onion and sauté until it is translucent, about 5 minutes. Add the cumin and garlic. Stir to combine and cook 1 minute more.

4. Add the chipotle chile in adobo sauce, roasted poblano peppers, pork, stock, and oregano. Bring to a low simmer, then cover and let cook 20 minutes.

Continued

Pork and Poblano Stew *Continued*

1 small cilantro
  bunch, chopped

½ cup pepitas

½ cup sour cream

5. Add the sweet potato and corn. Simmer 20 minutes, until the sweet potato is fully tender.

6. To serve, ladle into bowls and stir in the cilantro. Top with the pepitas and sour cream. Serve immediately.

Recipe tip: Use caution when roasting poblanos in the broiler. Long-handled tongs will be your friend here, as will a kitchen mitt to protect your hands and wrists. If using a gas stovetop instead, place the poblanos over the flame and use long-handled tongs to rotate them to evenly roast. Repeat the other steps as directed for cooling and deseeding the peppers after roasting.

Per serving: Calories: 460; Fat: 27g; Protein: 29g; Cholesterol: 85mg; Sodium: 430mg; Carbohydrates: 27g; Fiber: 5g

Hungarian Paprika and Pork Stew

SERVES 4 to 6 | **PREP TIME** 10 MINUTES | **COOK TIME** 40 MINUTES

This recipe features a sweet (versus smoky) flavor of paprika. Look for Hungarian or Spanish paprika when shopping. A heavily spiced stew like this can be an easy way to entice us to eat more vegetables, a key part of an anti-inflammatory diet. You may serve this stew over rice or noodles.

GLUTEN-FREE,
QUICK PREP

1 pork tenderloin, trimmed
   and cut into 1-inch cubes

1½ tablespoons sweet
   paprika, divided

Salt

Black pepper

2 tablespoons olive
   oil, divided

1 medium Vidalia
   onion, diced

10 ounces white or baby
   bella mushrooms,
   washed and sliced

2 garlic cloves, minced

½ teaspoon dried thyme

1 (14.5-ounce) can diced
   tomatoes, with juices

1. Toss the pork in a bowl with half of the paprika, salt, and pepper. Heat 1 tablespoon of olive oil in a large heavy-bottomed skillet over medium-high heat. Add the pork and cook, turning frequently to brown all sides, about 5 minutes.

2. Transfer the pork to a dish to keep warm. Add the remaining 1 tablespoon of olive oil, along with the onion. Cook 10 minutes, until the onion begins to brown and caramelize, then add the mushrooms, garlic, remaining paprika, and thyme. Cook another 2 minutes.

3. Add the tomatoes and stock. Bring to a simmer and cook, uncovered, for 10 minutes. Add the peas and transfer the cooked pork back to the stew. Cover, then cook another 10 minutes.

4. Remove from the heat and stir in the sour cream. Serve immediately.

Continued

2 cups *Chicken Stock*
  (page 25)

1 cup *frozen sweet peas*

½ cup *sour cream*

Ingredient tip: If a thicker consistency is preferred reduce the amount of chicken stock by 1 cup or increase cooking time to allow liquid to reduce.

Ingredient tip: The bulk section can be helpful when you need large quantities of a spice, but it's also helpful in instances like this when you may be purchasing only a small amount for one recipe.

Per serving: Calories: 380; Fat: 17g; Protein: 36g; Cholesterol: 100mg; Sodium: 570mg; Carbohydrates: 21g; Fiber: 4g

Asian Pork Soup with Cabbage

SERVES 6 | PREP TIME 10 MINUTES | **COOK TIME** 30 MINUTES

Napa cabbage (or Chinese cabbage) is an undercelebrated vegetable outside of its use in kimchi. It has a crisp texture and is related to other vegetables in the Brassica family such as broccoli, bok choy, and cauliflower. Use any remaining napa cabbage as a topper for other soups, stews, or tacos, or mix it into salads.

DAIRY-FREE,
QUICK PREP

2 tablespoons olive oil

1 pound pork
   tenderloin, cubed

Salt

Black pepper

10 ounces shiitake
   mushrooms, sliced

3 garlic cloves, minced

6 cups Chicken Broth
   (page 24)

2 tablespoons dry sherry

2 tablespoons low-
   sodium soy sauce

½ teaspoon ground
   ginger or 2 teaspoons
   grated fresh ginger

¼ teaspoon red
   pepper flakes

½ napa cabbage head, thinly
   sliced (about 2 cups)

2 scallions, thinly sliced

1. Heat the olive oil in a large stockpot or Dutch oven over medium-high heat. Season the pork with salt and pepper, then add the pork to the skillet and sear on all sides, about 5 minutes.

2. Add the mushrooms and garlic to the pot and stir to combine. Cook for 2 to 3 minutes until the mushrooms release their liquid and the garlic becomes fragrant.

3. Stir in the broth, sherry, soy sauce, ginger, and red pepper flakes. Bring to a boil, then reduce to a simmer. Cook 8 to 10 minutes, until the pork is fully cooked and tender.

4. Add the cabbage and scallions, then remove from the heat. Serve immediately.

Ingredient tip: If you don't have dry sherry, look for rice vinegar. Adjust according to your tastes, adding a conservative amount at first and adding more if needed.

Per serving: Calories: 190; Fat: 8g; Protein: 23g; Cholesterol: 50mg; Sodium: 370mg; Carbohydrates: 8g; Fiber: 2g

Moroccan Lamb Stew

SERVES 8 | **PREP TIME** 15 MINUTES | **COOK TIME** 1 HOUR 45 MINUTES

Lamb is a celebrated meat throughout the Mediterranean. As a nutrient-packed powerhouse, lamb is a source of healthy, unsaturated fats. Nearly 40 percent of the fat in lean lamb is heart-healthy monounsaturated fat. This Moroccan stew is sweet, spicy, and fragrant, warming the soul.

DAIRY-FREE,
GLUTEN-FREE

1½ pounds lamb shoulder,
   in 1-inch cubes

1 teaspoon ground cumin

1 teaspoon ground ginger

½ teaspoon ground
   cinnamon

¼ teaspoon cayenne pepper

3 tablespoons olive
   oil, divided

1 medium onion, diced

4 garlic cloves, minced

2 large carrots, cut into
   ½-inch rounds

1½ cups cubed
   butternut squash

1 (28-ounce) can fire-roasted
   diced tomatoes, with juices

1 (15-ounce) can chickpeas,
   drained and rinsed

Juice and zest of half
   of an orange

¼ cup cubed dried apricots

¼ cup raisins

2 cups Beef Stock (page 26)

1. In a medium bowl combine the lamb, cumin, ginger, cinnamon, and cayenne pepper and coat the lamb with the spices.

2. In a large pot, heat 2 tablespoons of olive oil over medium-high heat. Working in batches, add the lamb and brown on all sides, about 5 minutes per batch. Remove the lamb with a slotted spoon and transfer to a plate.

3. Turn down the heat to medium and heat the remaining 1 tablespoon of olive oil. Add the onion and sauté until it is translucent, about 5 minutes. Add the garlic and cook until fragrant, 1 to 2 minutes. Add the carrots and squash, and cook for 5 minutes, until the vegetables begin to soften.

4. Add the browned lamb, tomatoes, chickpeas, orange juice and zest, apricots, raisins, stock, cinnamon stick, and bay leaf.

5. Bring the stew to a boil, stirring gently to scrape all the brown bits from the bottom of the pot. Reduce the heat to low, cover, and simmer until the lamb is tender, 1 to 1½ hours, stirring every 20 minutes.

6. Season with salt and pepper to taste. Garnish with the parsley and mint.

1 cinnamon stick

1 bay leaf

Salt

Black pepper

1 tablespoon chopped fresh
 parsley, for garnish

2 tablespoons sliced fresh
 mint leaves, for garnish

Ingredient tip: Beans, like chickpeas, are pantry staples in many Moroccan homes. They're nutritious, budget friendly, and truly delicious when prepared in Moroccan stews, couscous, soups, and purées.

Ingredient tip: Use the fresh cut butternut squash or opt for frozen to shortcut your prep time.

Per serving: Calories: 310; Fat: 13g; Protein: 22g; Cholesterol: 55mg; Sodium: 570mg; Carbohydrates: 28g; Fiber: 5g

Chickpea Lamb Shawarma Stew

SERVES 8 | **PREP TIME** 15 MINUTES | **COOK TIME** 30 MINUTES

Shawarma is a heavily seasoned roasted meat, cooked on a revolving spit and shaved for serving in sandwiches. Enjoy these vibrant flavors in a bowl of soup. Create your own shawarma seasoning blend with spices you probably already have in your pantry!

GLUTEN-FREE

For shawarma spice mix

1½ teaspoons garam masala

1 teaspoon ground cumin

½ teaspoon cayenne pepper

¼ teaspoon ground cinnamon

1 teaspoon salt

½ teaspoon black pepper

For the stew

2 tablespoons olive oil

1 medium onion, chopped

4 garlic cloves, minced

1 pound ground lamb

2 tablespoons tomato paste

1 (28-ounce) can crushed tomatoes

2 cups Chicken Stock (page 25)

2 large carrots, peeled and diced

1 (15-ounce) can chickpeas, drained and rinsed

To make the shawarma spice mix

In a small bowl, combine the garam masala, cumin, cayenne pepper, cinnamon, salt, and pepper. Mix and set aside.

To make the stew

1. In a large pot, heat the olive oil over medium-high heat. Add the onion and sauté until it is translucent, about 5 minutes. Add the garlic and cook until fragrant, 1 to 2 minutes.

2. Add the lamb and tomato paste. Cook until the lamb is no longer pink, about 2 to 3 minutes, breaking it up into pieces with a wooden spoon. Add the spice mixture and stir to combine.

3. Add the crushed tomatoes, stock, carrots, and chickpeas. Bring to a simmer, cover, and cook for 15 to 20 minutes, until the carrots are tender.

4. Add the Swiss chard, turn off the heat, and cover. Let the residual heat wilt the Swiss chard before serving.

5. Season with salt and pepper to taste. Top with Greek yogurt and cilantro, if using.

2 cups chopped stemmed
   Swiss chard

Salt

Black pepper

Plain Greek yogurt,
   chopped cilantro, for
   topping (optional)

Ingredient tip: On average, a 3-ounce portion of cooked lamb provides 92 percent of the daily value of vitamin B12. Found only in animal products, vitamin B12 supports many important metabolic functions.

Make it a meal: Serve with whole-wheat couscous or whole-grain pita bread for a full meal.

Per serving: Calories: 310; Fat: 19g; Protein: 16g; Cholesterol: 45mg; Sodium: 710mg; Carbohydrates: 21g; Fiber: 5g

Instant Pot Oxtail Stew

SERVES 6 | **PREP TIME** 15 MINUTES | **COOK TIME** 1 HOUR 20 MINUTES

Oxtail, also known as cow tail, is rich in connective tissue and collagen, making any kind of stew or soup extremely flavorful and satisfying. Never tried oxtail before? Think braised beef short ribs or shanks, but with even more flavor. As with most tough cuts, oxtail ordinarily requires a very long cooking time, but with an Instant Pot or pressure cooker, this delicious stew can be done within an hour.

2 pounds oxtail

Salt

Black pepper

2 tablespoons olive oil, divided

3 shallots, chopped

3 garlic cloves, minced

1 tablespoon butter

2 tablespoons flour

2 tablespoons tomato paste

6 cups Beef Stock (page 26)

2 bay leaves

1 thyme sprig

1 rosemary sprig

½ teaspoon red pepper flakes

1 cup pearl onions

2 medium carrots, peeled and sliced

1 pound potatoes, chopped

2 tablespoons chopped fresh parsley

1. Season the oxtail liberally with salt and pepper. Set the pressure cooker to sauté mode and add olive oil. Brown the oxtail on all sides, about 10 minutes. Remove the oxtail and set aside.

2. Add the shallots and garlic and sauté until translucent, about 5 minutes. Add the butter and flour and cook for 3 to 4 minutes until the flour absorbs the butter and forms a roux. Add the tomato paste and stir to coat the vegetables.

3. Return the oxtail to the pressure cooker. Add the stock, bay leaves, thyme, rosemary, and red pepper flakes. Stir to make sure everything is combined. Lock the lid and set to manual high pressure for 40 minutes. (Your appliance may also have "meat/stew" setting, which may be used for this recipe.)

4. When the cooking cycle ends, release the steam and remove the lid. Skim off any excess fat accumulated at the top. Add the pearl onions, carrots, and potatoes. Set on high for another 10 minutes to cook the vegetables. When the cooking cycle ends, release the steam and remove the lid.

5. Add the parsley. Season with salt and pepper to taste.

Ingredient tip: Can't find pearl onions in the produce section? They often have frozen and peeled pearl onions in the freezer section.

Ingredient tip: As the oxtail is cooking in the stew, the collagen from the bones is released, creating a nutrient-dense broth. The nutrients extracted from beef bones contain amino acids like glycine and glutamine that aid digestion and promote gut health.

Per serving: Calories: 390; Fat: 18g; Protein: 31g; Cholesterol: 110mg; Sodium: 720mg; Carbohydrates: 27g; Fiber: 3g

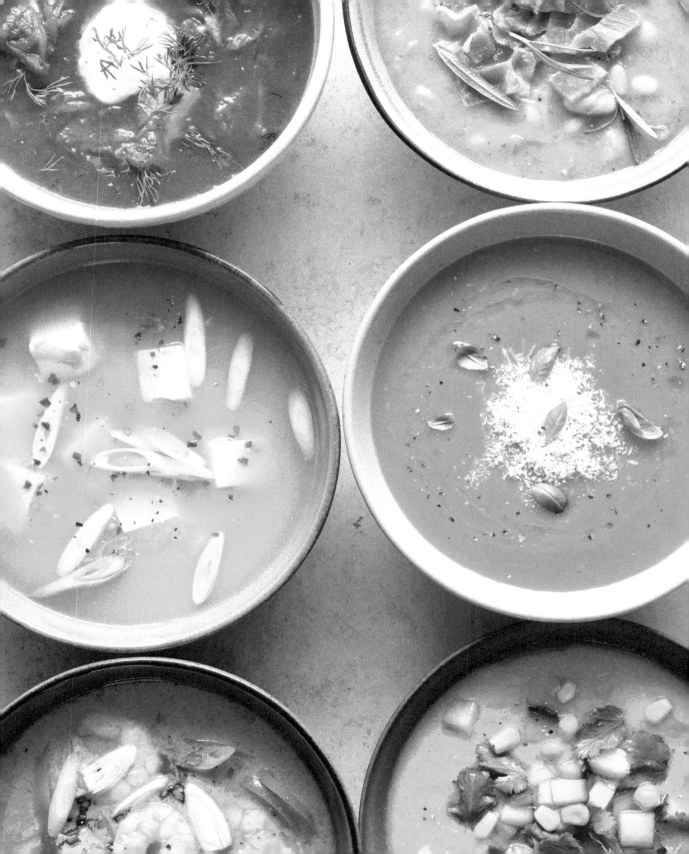

MEASUREMENT CONVERSIONS

VOLUME EQUIVALENTS (LIQUID)

US STANDARD	US STANDARD (OUNCES)	METRIC (APPROXIMATE)
2 tablespoons	1 fl. oz.	30 mL
¼ cup	2 fl. oz.	60 mL
½ cup	4 fl. oz.	120 mL
1 cup	8 fl. oz.	240 mL
1½ cups	12 fl. oz.	355 mL
2 cups or 1 pint	16 fl. oz.	475 mL
4 cups or 1 quart	32 fl. oz.	1 L
1 gallon	128 fl. oz.	4 L

OVEN TEMPERATURES

FAHRENHEIT	CELSIUS (APPROXIMATE)
250°F	120°C
300°F	150°C
325°F	165°C
350°F	180°C
375°F	190°C
400°F	200°C
425°F	220°C
450°F	230°C

VOLUME EQUIVALENTS (DRY)

US STANDARD	METRIC (APPROXIMATE)
⅛ teaspoon	0.5 mL
¼ teaspoon	1 mL
½ teaspoon	2 mL
¾ teaspoon	4 mL
1 teaspoon	5 mL
1 tablespoon	15 mL
¼ cup	59 mL
⅓ cup	79 mL
½ cup	118 mL
⅔ cup	156 mL
¾ cup	177 mL
1 cup	235 mL
2 cups or 1 pint	475 mL
3 cups	700 mL
4 cups or 1 quart	1 L

WEIGHT EQUIVALENTS

US STANDARD	METRIC (APPROXIMATE)
½ ounce	15 g
1 ounce	30 g
2 ounces	60 g
4 ounces	115 g
8 ounces	225 g
12 ounces	340 g
16 ounces or 1 pound	455 g

INDEX

ACKNOWLEDGMENTS

We'd like to thank the team at Callisto Media and Rockridge Press for the guidance and oversight in navigating this project and supporting us in bringing these healing soups to those who crave them.

Cara & Julie

ABOUT THE AUTHORS

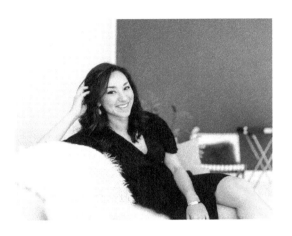

CARA HARBSTREET, MS, RD, LD, is a registered dietitian and nationally recognized food and nutrition expert. She attended Southeast Missouri State University and completed her master of science and dietetic internship at the University of Kansas Medical Center. She owns and operates Street Smart Nutrition, which provides nutrition coaching and counseling to clients in Kansas City and beyond.

Cara is passionate about helping people rediscover joy in eating deeply nourishing foods without restriction or fear. She is the author of *The Pescatarian Cookbook: The Essential Kitchen Companion* and *Healthy Eating for Life: An Intuitive Eating Workbook to Stop Dieting Forever.*

She resides in Kansas City and enjoys traveling, experimenting in the kitchen, and exploring local restaurants. You can connect with her at streetsmartnutrition.com, as well as on social media.

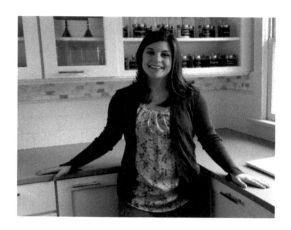

JULIE HARRINGTON, RD, is a registered dietitian and chef. She obtained a bachelor of science degree in culinary nutrition from Johnson & Wales University. She went on to complete her dietetic internship at the College of Saint Elizabeth.

Cooking has always given Julie joy because of its powerful ability to connect people. As a nationally recognized food and nutrition expert, Julie's passion is to educate others and give them the tools they need to build confidence in the kitchen.

She is the creator and owner of Julie Harrington Consulting LLC at julieharringtonrd.com, where she shares nutrition expertise and showcases simple and delicious recipes.

She resides in New Jersey with her official recipe taste-tester and soon-to-be husband, Adrian, and their corgi, Wally.

CPSIA information can be obtained
at www.ICGtesting.com
Printed in the USA
BVHW052312300819
557299BV00002B/2